MRCOG PART
PRACTICE EXAMS

MRCOG PART I PRACTICE EXAMS

Paul Hilton MD BS MRCOG
Senior Lecturer in Obstetrics and Gynaecology, University of Newcastle upon Tyne and Honorary Consultant, Newcastle Health Authority.

Keith A Godfrey MBChB MRCOG
Consultant Obstetrician and Gynaecologist, Sunderland District General Hospital.

David Ireland MD BChir MA MRCOG
First Assistant in Obstetrics and Gynaecology, University of Newcastle upon Tyne and Honorary Senior Registrar, Northern Regional Health Authority.

PASTEST SERVICE
KNUTSFORD
CHESHIRE
ENGLAND

© 1986 PASTEST SERVICE
Cranford Lodge
Bexton Road
KNUTSFORD, Cheshire WA16 0ED
Tel: 0565-755226

Reprinted 1989, 1991

British Library Cataloguing in Publication Data

Hilton, P.
MRCOG Part I practice exams : 5 practice exams for MRCOG candidates all with correct answers and teaching explanations.
1. Gynaecology—Examinations, questions, etc.
2. Obstetrics—Examinations, questions, etc.
I. Title   II. Godfrey, K. A.   III. Ireland, D.
618′.076   RG111
ISBN 0-906896-25-8

Text prepared by Turner Associates, Knutsford, Cheshire
Phototypeset by Communitype, Leicester
Printed and bound in Great Britain by
Biddles Ltd, Guildford and King's Lynn

CONTENTS

EXAMINATION TECHNIQUE

Multiple Choice Questions are the most consistent, reproducible and internally reliable method we have of testing re-call of factual knowledge. Yet there is evidence that they are able to test more than simple factual re-call; reasoning ability and an understanding of basic facts, principles and concepts can also be assessed. A good MCQ paper will discriminate accurately between candidates on the basis of their knowledge of the topics being tested. It must be emphasised that the most important function of an MCQ paper of the type used in the MRCOG Part 1, is to rank candidates accurately and fairly according to their performance in that paper. Accurate ranking is the key phrase; this means that all MCQ examinations of this type are, in a sense, competitive.

Technique
The safest way to pass MRCOG Part 1 is to know the answers to all of the questions, but it is equally important to be able to transfer this knowledge accurately onto the answer sheet. All too often, candidates suffer through an inability to organise their time, through failure to read the instructions carefully or through failure to read and understand the questions. First of all you must allocate your time with care. There are two examination papers covering the syllabus in six topics: anatomy and embryology; endocrinology; microbiology and pharmacology; physiology and genetics; pathology and immunology; biochemistry. In each paper there are 60 questions (each of 5 parts) to be completed in 2 hours; this means 2 minutes per question or 10 questions in 20 minutes. Make sure that you are getting through the exam at least at this pace, or, if possible, a little quicker, thus allowing time at the end for revision and a re-think on some of the items that you have deferred.

You must read the question (both stem and items) carefully. You should be quite clear that you know what you are being asked to do. Once you know this, you should indicate your responses by marking the paper boldly, correctly and clearly. Take great care not to mark the wrong ovals and think very carefully before making a mark on the answer sheet.

Regard each item as being independent of each other item, each refers to a specific quantum of knowledge. The item (or the stem and the item taken together) make up a statement. You are required to indicate whether you regard this statement as 'True' or 'False' and you are also able to indicate 'Don't know'. Look only at a single statement when answering, disregard all the other statements presented in the question. They have nothing to do with the item you are concentrating on.

Marking your answer sheets
The answer sheet will be read by an automatic document reader, which

transfers the information it reads to a computer. It must therefore be filled out in accordance with the instructions. You must first fill in your name on the answer sheet, and then fill in your examination number. It is critical that this is filled in correctly.

As you go through the questions, you can either mark your answers immediately on the answer sheet, or you can mark them in the question book first, transferring them to the answer sheets at the end. If you adopt the second approach, you must take great care not to run out of time, since you will not be allowed extra time to transfer marks to the answer sheet from the question book. The answer sheet must always be marked neatly and carefully according to the instructions given. Careless marking is probably one of the commonest causes of rejection of answer sheets by the document reader. For although the computer operator will do his best to interpret correctly the answer you intended, and will then correct the sheet accordingly, the procedure introduces a possible new source of error. You are, of course, at liberty to change your mind by erasing your original selection and selecting a new one. In this event, your erasure should be carefully, neatly, and completely carried out.

Try to leave time to go over your answers again before the end, in particular going back over any difficult questions that you wish to think about in more detail. At the same time, you can check that you have marked the answer sheet correctly. However, repeated review of your answers may in the end be counter-productive, since answers that you were originally confident were absolutely correct, often look rather less convincing at a second, third or fourth perusal. In this situation, first thoughts are usually best and too critical a revision might lead you into a state of confusion.

To guess or not to guess
Do not mark at random. Candidates are frequently uncertain whether or not to guess the answer. However, a clear distinction must be made between a genuine guess (i.e. tales for True, heads for False) and a process of reasoning by which you attempt to work out an answer that is not immediately apparent by using first principles and drawing on your knowledge and experience. Genuine guesses should not be made. You might be lucky, but if you are totally ignorant of the answer, there is an equal chance that you will be wrong and thus lose marks. This is not a chance that is worth taking, and you should not hesitate to indicate 'Don't know' if this genuinely and honestly expresses your view.

Although you should not guess, you should not give in too easily. What you are doing is to increase as much as possible the odds that the answer you are going to give is the correct one, even though you are not 100%

certain that this is the case. Take time to think, therefore, drawing on first principles and reasoning power, and delving into your memory stores. Do not, however, spend an inordinate amount of time on a single item that is puzzling you. Leave it, and, if you have time, return to it. If you are 'fairly certain' that you know the right answer or have been able to work it out, it is reasonable to mark the answer sheet accordingly. There is a difference between being 'fairly certain' (odds better than 50:50 that you are right) and totally ignorant (where any response would be a guess). The phrase 'MCQ technique' is often mentioned, and is usually used to refer specifically to this question of 'guessing' and 'Don't know'. Careful thought and reasoning ability, as well as honesty, are all involved in so-called 'technique', but the best way to increase the odds that you know the right answers to the questions, is to have a sound basic knowledge of medicine and its specialties.

Trust the examiners
Do try to trust the Examiners. Accept each question at its face value, and do not look for hidden meanings, catches and ambiguities. Multiple choice questions are not designed to trick or confuse you, they are designed to test your knowledge of medicine. Don't look for problems that aren't there – the obvious meaning of a statement is the correct one and the one that you should read. Candidates often try to calculate their score as they go through the paper; their theory is that if they reach a certain score they should then be safe in indicating 'Don't know' for any items that they have left blank without needing to take the trouble to think out answers. This approach is not to be recommended. No candidate can be certain what score he will need to achieve to obtain a pass in the examination, and everyone will overestimate the score he thinks he has obtained by answering questions confidently. The best approach is to answer every question honestly and to make every possible effort to work out the answers to more difficult questions, leaving the 'Don't know' option to indicate exactly what it means. In other words, your aim should always be to obtain the highest possible score on the MCQ paper.

To repeat the four most important points of technique:

(1) Read the question carefully and be sure you understand it.
(2) Mark your responses clearly, correctly and accurately.
(3) Use reasoning to work out answers, but if you do not know the answer and cannot work it out, indicate 'Don't know'.
(4) The best way to obtain a good mark is to have as wide a knowledge as possible of the topics being tested in the examination.

MCQ INSTRUCTIONS

In order to help MRCOG Part 1 candidates revise for this difficult examination we have tried to follow as closely a possible the content and format of the official examination. Each question has an answer and teaching explanation which should provide a good basis for successful revision.

We suggest that you work on each set of 60 multiple choice questions as though it were a real examination. In other words time yourself to spend no more than 2 hours on each practice exam and do not obtain help from books, notes or persons while working on each test. Plan to take this practice exam at a time when you will be undisturbed for a minimum of 2 hours. Choose a well lit location free from distractions, keep your desk clear of other books or papers, have a clock or watch clearly visible with a rubber and 2 well sharpened grade B pencils to hand.

As you work through each question in this book be sure and mark a T or F (True or False) against the A...B...C...D...E... answer space below each question. If you do not know the answer then leave the answer space blank. Thus, when you have completed the paper you can mark your own answers with the aid of the answers and explanations given at the end of the book. Do not be tempted to look at the questions before sitting down to take each test as this will not then represent a mock exam.

When you have finished an exam be sure to go back over your answers until the 2 hours are over. When your time is up you can then mark your answers and study the teaching explanations carefully so as to learn from your mistakes. Give yourself +1 for every correct answer, -1 for every incorrect answer and 0 for an unanswered (don't know) question. Put a mark clearly in the book wherever you put a wrong answer and this will help you with your final revision as the official exam grows near.

Good luck with your revision.

PRACTICE EXAM 1

60 Questions : time allowed 2 hours.
Indicate your answers (T or F) in the space provided.

1   Prolactin

A   is structurally related to human placental lactogen (HPL)
B   is secreted by basophil cells of the anterior pituitary
C   is increased in the circulation after section of the pituitary stalk
D   is secreted in reduced amounts in patients taking chlorpromazine
E   can only be measured by bioassay

Your answers: A.......B.......C.......D.......E.......

2   The following renal changes are typical of normal pregnancy:

A   increased glomerular filtration rate
B   decreased excretion of urate
C   increased excretion of folate
D   increased excretion of glucose
E   ureteric dilatation

Your answers: A.......B.......C.......D.......E.......

3   In the autonomic nervous system

A   acetylcholine is the mediator at all synapses betwen pre- and post- ganglionic nerves
B   pseudo cholinesterase is localised at nerve endings
C   strychnine blocks the action of inhibitory interneurones in the spinal cord
D   adrenaline is the mediator of activity at most post-ganglionic sympathetic nerve endings
E   dopaminergic neurones are present in sympathetic ganglia

Your answers: A.......B.......C.......D.......E.......

4   The following statements about haemostasis are correct:

A   tissue thromboplastin activates factor VII
B   plasmin converts fibrin polymers to insoluble fibrin
C   in small blood vessels platelet aggregation follows fibrin deposition
D   thrombasthenia is the term used to describe platelet deficiency
E   prothrombin is vitamin K-dependent

Your answers: A.......B.......C.......D.......E.......

1

5   During exercise

A   pH increases
B   the dissociation curve for haemoglobin is shifted to the right
C   diastolic blood pressure rises
D   stroke volume decreases
E   body temperature rises

Your answers: A.......B.......C.......D.......E.......

6   The following physiological measurements are increased in normal healthy pregnancy:

A   pulse rate
B   serum colloid osmotic pressure
C   glomerular filtration rate
D pCO_2
E   gastric emptying time

Your answers: A.......B.......C.......D.......E.......

7   The following changes in blood pressure control have occurred by the second trimester of normal pregnancy:

A   peripheral resistance is increased
B   plasma renin activity is decreased
C   cardiac output is unchanged
D   aldosterone excretion is increased
E   myocardial contractility is increased

Your answers: A.......B.......C.......D.......E.......

8   In the bladder

A   intravesical pressure increases linearly with intravesical urine volume
B   the first urge to void is felt at a volume of 500 ml
C   normal micturition is dependent on an intact sympathetic nerve supply
D   the urge to void is only felt after the detrusor pressure exceeds 20 cm water
E   after spinal transection in the thoracic region the voiding reflex may return

Your answers: A.......B.......C.......D.......E.......

2

9   During pregnancy

A   glycosuria is an effective test of carbohydrate intolerance
B   fasting plasma glucose concentration is decreased
C   fasting plasma insulin concentration is decreased
D   the oral glucose tolerance test alters with advancing gestation
E   two hours after an oral glucose load, plasma insulin concentration should have returned to fasting levels

Your answers: A.......B.......C.......D.......E.......

10   The amnion

A   is surrounded by the chorion
B   is derived from the blastocyst
C   in a dizygous (binovular) twin pregnancy is separated from its fellow by the chorion
D   covers the fetal surface of the placenta
E   separates from the decidua in the third stage of labour

Your answers: A.......B.......C.......D.......E.......

11   Prostaglandins

A   are small molecular weight polypeptides
B   are chemically related to thromboxanes
C   have been clearly shown to be responsible for luteolysis in man
D   inhibit the secretion of renin
E   are produced in the seminal vesicles of man

Your answers: A.......B.......C.......D.......E.......

12   Human milk

A   contains less than 4% protein
B   is equal to cows' milk in fat content
C   has a higher sodium concentration than human colostrum
D   is a poor source of iron for the neonate
E   is a poor source of B vitamins for the neonate

Your answers: A.......B.......C.......D.......E.......

13 **The following statements about vitamins are correct:**

A   most vitamins can be synthesised in adequate amounts in the body
B   vitamin K is water soluble
C   deficiency of pyridoxine (vitamin B6) can cause convulsions
D   naturally occurring folate contains a single glutamic acid residue
E   excessive vitamin D intake may cause renal failure

Your answers: A.......B.......C.......D.......E.......

14 **Which of the following spinal roots contribute to the pudendal nerve:**

A   L5
B   S1
C   S2
D   S3
E   S4

Your answers: A.......B.......C.......D.......E.......

15 **In diabetes mellitus**

A   the appetite is increased
B   glucagon secretion is increased
C   intestinal absorption of glucose is enhanced
D   glucose uptake by skeletal muscle is reduced
E   glucocorticoid secretion is increased in the well-controlled patient

Your answers: A.......B.......C.......D.......E.......

16 **Human placental lactogen (HPL)**

A   closely resembles pituitary growth hormone
B   is detectable during pregnancy 35 days after the LH peak
C   decreases the availability of glucose to the fetus
D   augments fat metabolism
E   is decreased in twin pregnancies

Your answers: A.......B.......C.......D.......E.......

17 **The following structures support the uterus:**

A   the round ligaments
B   the utero-sacral ligaments
C   the broad ligaments
D   the transverse cervical (cardinal) ligaments
E   the bulbocavernosus

Your answers: A.......B.......C.......D.......E.......

18 **The following statements about plasma lipids are correct:**

A   chylomicra are not normally present in the plasma of a person who has fasted 12 hours or more
B   in the fasting state circulating free fatty acids are adsorbed to plasma albumin
C   high density lipoproteins contain most of the circulating cholesterol
D   the low density lipoprotein fraction corresponds to the β lipoprotein fraction on electrophoresis
E   plasma free fatty acid concentration is reduced in the fasting state

Your answers: A.......B.......C.......D.......E.......

19 **The following organisms may cause aseptic meningitis:**

A   Lassa virus
B   respiratory syncytial virus
C   mumps virus
D   influenza virus
E   human genital wart virus

Your answers: A.......B.......C.......D.......E.......

20 **The following arise from Wolffian remnants:**

A   the epoophoron
B   the processus vaginalis
C   the paroophoron
D   the round ligament
E   Gartner's duct

Your answers: A.......B.......C.......D.......E.......

21   In normal pregnancy

A   there are equal increases in the excretion of oestrone, oestradiol and oestriol
B   serum HCG concentration rises to a peak at 20 weeks gestation
C   there is a reduced aldosterone secretion
D   androgen excretion is reduced
E   there is an increase in serum protein-bound iodine

Your answers: A.......B.......C.......D.......E.......

22   Which of the following are pathogenic Gram-positive spore-bearing bacteria growing readily under aerobic conditions:

A   Bacillus anthracis
B   Clostridium welchii
C   Pseudomonas aeruginosa
D   Corynebacterium diptheriae
E   Clostridium botulinum

Your answers: A.......B.......C.......D.......E.......

23   In human genetics

A   the total number of chromosomes in both normal males and females is 46
B   in the female, the sex chromosomes are XY
C   chromatic positive cells (Barr body present) are characteristic of normal males
D   the sexual differentiation of the fetal gonads occurs about the 7th week
E   the Y chromosome determines the development of the ovary

Your answers: A.......B.......C.......D.......E.......

24   The following progestogens are derived from testosterone:

A   ethynodiol
B   megestrol
C   norgestrel
D   chlormadinone
E   norethisterone

Your answers: A.......B.......C.......D.......E.......

25   The following cytotoxic drugs are alkylating agents:

A   anthracycline
B   chlorambucil
C   6-mercaptopurine
D   cyclophosphamide
E   vinblastine

Your answers: A.......B.......C.......D.......E.......

26   The following statements are correct:

A   insulin promotes the uptake of glucose by muscle cells
B   glucose-6-phosphatase occurs in muscle but not in liver
C   adrenaline promotes the breakdown of hepatic glycogen
D   lactate is the end product of the aerobic metabolism of glucose
E   insulin is secreted by the alpha cells of the Islets of Langerhans

Your answers: A.......B.......C.......D.......E.......

27   The following statements which apply to aerobic glycolysis are correct:

A   glucose is broken down to form lactic acid
B   it requires components of the respiratory chain
C   it takes place in mitochondria
D   oxygen reacts directly with glucose
E   the energy produced is stored as ATP

Your answers: A.......B.......C.......D.......E.......

28   During mitosis

A   the last phase is telophase
B   crossing over occurs at prophase
C   anaphase lag may occur
D   prophase is very prolonged
E   replication occurs

Your answers: A.......B.......C.......D.......E.......

29   **Absorption or reabsorption take place in the**

    A   oesophagus
    B   first part of the duodenum
    C   colon
    D   ureter
    E   collecting tubules of the kidney

Your answers: A.......B.......C.......D.......E.......

30   **The cervix of the uterus**

    A   undergoes cyclical changes during the menstrual cycle
    B   sheds its lining at menstruation
    C   has a lining of columnar epithelium in its canal
    D   may have glands opening onto its vaginal surface
    E   has peritoneum on the posterior surface of its supravaginal part

Your answers: A.......B.......C.......D.......E.......

31   **The following changes occur during normal pregnancy:**

    A   spider angiomata
    B   raised serum cholesterol concentration
    C   raised serum alkaline phosphatase
    D   increased serum transaminase
    E   prolonged prothrombin time

Your answers: A.......B.......C.......D.......E.......

32   **The menopause**

    A   occurs earlier than formerly
    B   is associated with increased bone density
    C   is associated with an increase in vaginal acidity
    D   is associated with a rise in oestradiol and a fall in oestrone
    E   is associated with greater shrinkage of the uterine body than of the cervix

Your answers: A.......B.......C.......D.......E.......

33   The rectum

A   is covered anteriorly by peritoneum along its whole length
B   has no taeniae coli
C   has appendices epipliocae
D   has a blood supply from the terminal branches of the superior mesenteric artery
E   has permanent transverse folds consisting of mucous membrane and circular smooth muscle

Your answers: A.......B.......C.......D.......E.......

34   The following are recessive conditions:

A   cystic fibrosis
B   phenylketonuria
C   thalassaemia
D   congenital pyloric stenosis
E   Hirschsprungs' disease

Your answers: A.......B.......C.......D.......E.......

35   The following statements relating to the small intestine are correct:

A   the small intestine becomes narrower throughout its course
B   circular folds (valves of Kerckring) are more frequent in the ileum than in the jejunum
C   villi are shorter in the jejunum than in the ileum
D   Brunner's glands are most frequent in the jejunum
E   Paneth cells are found only in the bases of the crypts of Lieberkuhn

Your answers: A.......B.......C.......D.......E.......

36   In the human placenta

A   the syncytiotrophoblast lies deep to the cytotrophoblast
B   iron is stored in trophoblast tissue
C   fibrinoid deposits are present during healthy pregnancies
D   placental septa develop from fetal mesoderm
E   the number of main stem villi (trunci chorii) remains constant throughout pregnancy

Your answers: A.......B.......C.......D.......E.......

9

37 In the kidney

A   the columns of Bertini contain cortical tissue
B   all nephrons have equally long loops of Henle
C   the afferent arteriole at the glomerulus has a thicker muscular wall than the efferent arteriole
D   the macula densa arises from the wall of the proximal convoluted tubule
E   the renal pelvis contains smooth muscle fibres

Your answers: A.......B.......C.......D.......E.......

38 The round ligament

A   is over 25 cm long
B   runs posterior to the obturator artery
C   is embryologically related to the ovarian ligament
D   passes lateral to the inferior epigastric artery
E   contains striated muscle fibres

Your answers: A.......B.......C.......D.......E.......

39 The following statements relating to the adrenal glands are correct:

A   the average weight of the normal adrenal gland in the adult is 1 gram
B   each gland is drained by three separate veins
C   the medulla is endodermal in origin
D   the zona reticularis of the cortex lies next to the medulla
E   aldosterone is produced by cells of the zona glomerulosa of the cortex

Your answers: A.......B.......C.......D.......E.......

40 The following statements relating to the histology of the skin are correct:

A   apocrine sweat glands are the most common in man
B   the arrectores pili muscles contribute to sebum release
C   in split-skin grafts only half of the thickness of the epidermis is removed
D   melanocytes synthesise the enzyme tyrosinase
E   corpuscles of Ruffini are receptors for touch

Your answers: A.......B.......C.......D.......E.......

41   As used in statistics, the median of a series of observations is the

A   sum total of values divided by the number of observations
B   centre value with the observations ranged in order from highest to lowest
C   value occurring most often
D   distance between the highest and lowest values
E   the square root of the standard deviation

Your answers: A.......B.......C.......D.......E.......

42   The following statements relating to the lesser sac of the peritoneum (omental bursa) are correct:

A   the sac lies anterior to the origin of the hepatic artery
B   the opening of the sac (foramen of Winslow) is posterior to the hepatic artery
C   the body of the stomach forms part of the posterior wall of the sac
D   the caudate lobe of the liver forms part of the superior boundary of the sac
E   the sac separates the transverse mesocolon from the mesentery

Your answers: A.......B.......C.......D.......E.......

43   The following are primary branches of the coeliac artery:

A   left gastric artery
B   right gastro-epiploic artery
C   gastro-duodenal artery
D   hepatic artery
E   splenic artery

Your answers: A.......B.......C.......D.......E.......

44   At the inguinal ligament

A   the femoral artery lies lateral to the femoral vein
B   the femoral nerve passes through the femoral ring
C   the pectineus muscle forms the posterior boundary of the femoral ring
D   the inferior epigastric artery runs lateral to the deep inguinal ring
E   the ilio-inguinal nerve passes through the inguinal canal

Your answers: A.......B.......C.......D.......E.......

45 The following are synovial joints:

A   symphysis pubis
B   sacro-iliac
C   sacro-coccygeal
D   lumbo-sacral
E   patello-femoral

Your answers: A.......B.......C.......D.......E.......

46 The following statements relating to nerves of the pelvis are correct:

A   the genito-femoral nerve arises from L1 and L2
B   the levator ani is in part supplied by the perineal nerve
C   the pudendal nerve lies just posterior to the sacro-tuberous ligament
D   the skin of the anal triangle is supplied by S1 and S2 fibres
E   the obturator nerve arises from the sacral plexus

Your answers: A.......B.......C.......D.......E.......

47 The following statements relating to the haemopoietic tissues are correct:

A   red marrow is present in the bones of the vault of the adult skull
B   sinusoids in marrow are lined by typical endothelial cells
C   lymphocytes are produced in bone marrow
D   the red cell nucleus is extruded at the polychromatophilic erythroblast stage
E   megakaryocytes are polyploid

Your answers: A.......B.......C.......D.......E.......

48 The following statements relating to *Clostridia* and clostridial infection are correct:

A   all *Clostridia* are anaerobes
B   *Cl. tetani* produces central spores
C   *Cl. perfringens* (*welchii*) is the only organism which causes gas gangrene
D   *Cl. perfringens* (*welchii*) must be actively treated when isolated from vaginal swabs
E   patients with tetanus must be barrier-nursed

Your answers: A.......B.......C.......D.......E.......

49   **The following statements relating to syphilis are correct:**

A   *Treponema pallidum* is a Gram-negative organism
B   the primary chancre usually appears within one week of exposure to infection
C   spirochaetes are distributed throughout the body at the time of appearance of the primary chancre
D   serology is positive in all cases of tertiary syphilis
E   the Wasserman reaction (WR) is specific for syphilis

Your answers: A.......B.......C.......D.......E.......

50   **Cytomegalovirus**

A   has infected over 60% of the adult population
B   is demonstrable in 0.5 to 1.5% of neonates
C   is an adenovirus
D   causes neonatal jaundice
E   is commonly present in the salivary glands

Your answers: A.......B.......C.......D.......E.......

51   **The following organisms commonly cause acute meningitis:**

A   *Haemophilus influenzae*
B   *Neisseria meningitidis*
C   *β haemolytic streptococcus*
D   *Staphylococcus albus*
E   *Diplococcus pneumoniae*

Your answers: A.......B.......C.......D.......E.......

52   **In the development of fetal sex organs**

A   the presence of ovaries is necessary for the development of the paramesonephric ducts
B   the pronephric duct degenerates as the mesonephros develops
C   ova originate outside the developing gonad
D   the vagina is formed entirely by invagination of the paramesonephric ducts
E   sexual differentiation of the external genitalia is complete before the 10th week of life

Your answers: A.......B.......C.......D.......E.......

53 **The following statements relating to the embryology of the pharynx are correct:**

A   the tympanic membrane is derived from the first pharyngeal pouch
B   the second pharyngeal arch develops into the mandible
C   the thymus develops from the second pharyngeal pouch
D   the anterior lobe of the pituitary gland develops from the third pharyngeal pouch
E   the foramen caecum is a remnant of the thyroglossal duct
Your answers: A.......B.......C.......D.......E.......

54 **The following statements about haemophilia are true:**

A   all sons of affected males will inherit the condition
B   half of the sons of a carrier female will inherit the condition
C   normal daughters cannot be born to a carrier female
D   the incidence of haemophilia in the daughters of an affected male (married to a normal female) will be one in four
E   if a carrier female marries an affected male, all of the offspring will inherit the haemophilia gene
Your answers: A.......B.......C.......D.......E.......

55 **The following statements concerning immunoglobulins are correct:**

A   these are all gamma-globulins
B   the five classes of immunoglobulins differ in their heavy polypeptide chains
C   IgG crosses the placental barrier
D   IgM is produced as the primary response to an antigen
E   IgE is predominantly found in the plasma
Your answers: A.......B.......C.......D.......E.......

56 **The following statements relate to the normal distribution:**

A   the mean and mode are equal
B   the median is one standard deviation below the mean
C   99.7% of the population lies within two standard deviations of the mean
D   the standard error of the mean is the variance divided by the square root of the number of observations
E   no other symmetrical distribution is possible
Your answers: A.......B.......C.......D.......E.......

57 Fetal heart rate

A   varies with gestational age
B   is not subject to parasympathetic activity before the 20th week of pregnancy
C   may accelerate with external head compression
D   increases as maternal temperature rises
E   accelerates in response to maternal ingestion of atropine sulphate
Your answers: A.......B.......C.......D.......E.......

58 The volume of amniotic fluid

A   is independent of fetal urine production
B   may be predicted accurately by ultrasound
C   is excessive in severe rhesus disease
D   increases following amniocentesis
E   is reduced in severe pre-eclampsia
Your answers: A.......B.......C.......D.......E.......

59 In women arterial blood pressure is elevated in association with the following:

A   age
B   parity
C   a sedentary occupation
D   obesity
E   a single gene mode of inheritance
Your answers: A.......B.......C.......D.......E.......

60 The characteristic cellular reaction found in tuberculosis usually includes

A   pus cells
B   siderocytes
C   foreign body giant cells
D   epithelioid cells
E   lymphocytes
Your answers: A.......B.......C.......D.......E.......

END OF EXAM 1

Go over your answers until the time is up. Then mark your answers according to the correct solutions given on page 76.

PRACTICE EXAM 2

60 Questions: time allowed 2 hours.
Indicate your answers (T or F) in the space provided.

1 Adequate sperm transport through the cervix is related to

A   changes in the cervical mucus at ovulation
B   anaerobic fructolysis within the semen
C   suction of semen into the uterus at intercourse
D   low pH within the cervical mucus
E   uterine anteversion

Your answers: A.......B.......C.......D.......E.......

2 Cervical mucus

A   contains immunoglobulins
B   contains proteinase inhibitors
C   will detect anovulatory infertility
D   will detect multiple pregnancy
E   does not exhibit ferning in the presence of blood

Your answers: A.......B.......C.......D.......E.......

3 Spermatogenesis

A   is a process requiring 110 ±5 days in the human male
B   requires both FSH and LH to stimulate sperm maturation
C   is associated with an increase in testosterone in the intertubu-
     lar tissue of the testis
D   is abnormal in a male with karyotype 47XXY
E   would cease in the absence of testosterone

Your answers: A.......B.......C.......D.......E.......

4 The erythrocyte sedimentation rate (ESR) is

A   more specific than serum C-reactive protein
B   usually raised in chronic inflammatory conditions
C   altered by age
D   of value in monitoring malignant disease
E   a reflection of serum cholesterol concentration

Your answers: A.......B.......C.......D.......E.......

5   Prostaglandins

A   are polypeptides found in prostatic fluid
B   induce rhythmic uterine contractions in a similar way to oxytocin
C   cause constipation in man
D   formation is inhibited by aspirin
E $PgF_2\alpha$ may cause bronchoconstriction

Your answers: A.......B.......C.......D.......E.......

6   The following factors positively influence high birth weight:

A   maternal growth hormone
B   prolonged pregnancy (>294 days)
C   fetal hyperinsulinaemia
D   primiparity
E   social class

Your answers: A.......B.......C.......D.......E.......

7   The following factors may cause a reduction of fetal growth potential:

A   altitude
B   maternal diabetes mellitus
C   cytomegalovirus infection
D   maternal stature
E   high pregnancy weight gain

Your answers: A.......B.......C.......D.......E.......

8   Renin

A   has a molecular weight of 65,000
B   is only produced in the kidney
C   is released when there is a rise in blood pressure
D   is released by decreased blood sodium concentration
E   falls in amount with a rise in plasma potassium

Your answers: A.......B.......C.......D.......E.......

9   In adult human blood

A   the monocyte is the largest of the circulating white cells
B   the mature lymphocyte has a basophilic cytoplasm
C   10% of the polymorphonuclear leucocytes in female subjects show a nuclear appendage
D   packed cell volume is less in women than in men
E   eosinophils constitute between 10 and 20% of the white cell count under normal conditions

Your answers: A.......B.......C.......D.......E.......

10   Human chorionic gonadotrophin (HCG)

A   has the biological properties of LH (luteinizing hormone)
B   can transform a normal cyclic corpus luteum into a pseudopregnant corpus luteum
C   is responsible for the onset of parturition
D   is detectable in maternal serum before implantation of the ovum
E   is significantly elevated in pre-eclampsia

Your answers: A.......B.......C.......D.......E.......

11   Human placental lactogen (HPL)

A   is a polypeptide hormone
B   is immunologically similar to human growth hormone
C   is produced by the syncytiotrophoblast
D   demonstrates a circadian rhythm
E   is of value in predicting fetal weight

Your answers: A.......B.......C.......D.......E.......

12   The following liver function changes occur in pregnancy:

A   serum alkaline phosphatase rises
B   serum cholesterol concentration falls
C   serum albumin concentration is reduced
D   serum globulin rises
E   transaminase concentration falls

Your answers: A.......B.......C.......D.......E.......

13   In the human fetus

A   the adrenal cortex contains a distinct cellular zone that disappears after birth
B   human growth hormone reaches its peak at birth
C   the pancreas responds to high levels of glucose
D   noradrenaline is produced solely by the adrenal medulla
E   the pituitary contains a pars intermedia

Your answers: A.......B.......C.......D.......E.......

14   Oxytocin is

A   a lipid hormone
B   synthesised in the anterior hypothalamic nuclei
C   released directly into the circulation from its site of production
D   an anti-diuretic
E   relatively inactive in early pregnancy

Your answers: A.......B.......C.......D.......E.......

15   In progesterone production and metabolism

A   only 10% of circulating hormone is free
B   the main source of the hormone in human pregnancy is the corpus luteum
C   cholesterol is a precursor
D   liver is the main site of degradation
E   the hormone causes increased excitability of the myometrium

Your answers: A.......B.......C.......D.......E.......

16   The following statements relating to thyroid function are correct:

A   TRH is a decapeptide
B   placental thyrotrophin is biochemically identical to pituitary TSH
C   the metabolic activity of T_3 is about four times that of T_4
D   5% of the circulating T_4 is free (not protein bound)
E   circulating TBG increases under the influence of oestrogens

Your answers: A.......B.......C.......D.......E.......

17   Progesterone

A   is natriuretic
B   requires oestrogen priming before it can demonstrate activity
      on the sexual organs
C   is synthesised in the adrenal gland
D   decreases uterine muscle contractility
E   is produced by arrhenoblastomas

Your answers: A.......B.......C.......D.......E.......

18   In the normal adult adrenal gland

A   aldosterone is produced in the zona glomerulosa
B   the cortex has a diurnal rhythm
C   aldosterone production is purely under control of ACTH
D   the zona glomerulosa forms the greater part of the cortex
E   cortisol production is under ACTH control

Your answers: A.......B.......C.......D.......E.......

19   The following drugs are anti-metabolites

A   cyclophosphamide
B   thiotepa
C   6-mercaptopurine
D   methotrexate
E   actinomycin

Your answers: A.......B.......C.......D.......E.......

20   Morphine

A   increases the concentration of alveolar pCO_2
B   dilates the pupils in man
C   causes orthostatic hypotension
D   causes a rise in intrabiliary duct pressure
E   is mainly excreted by the liver

Your answers: A.......B.......C.......D.......E.......

21   Prostaglandin E$_2$

A   is a uterine smooth muscle stimulant
B   is a protein hormone
C   production is inhibited by indomethacin
D   is released by platelets during blood coagulation
E   is an antidiuretic

Your answers: A.......B.......C.......D.......E.......

22   The following drugs have been shown to be harmful when given to a pregnant woman:

A   sulphadimidine
B   sodium amytal
C   tetracycline
D   chloramphenicol
E   ampicillin

Your answers: A.......B.......C.......D.......E.......

23   Histamine

A   causes local vasoconstriction in the skin
B   is found in mast cell granules
C   increases vascular permeability
D   is partially responsible for the triple response
E   stimulates gastric secretion

Your answers: A.......B.......C.......D.......E.......

24   The following carcinomas are common causes of secondary ovarian tumours:

A   breast
B   colon
C   cervix
D   lung
E   stomach

Your answers: A.......B.......C.......D.......E.......

25   The following tumours of the ovary are commonly endocrine secreting:

A   Brenner tumour
B   granulosa cell
C   arrhenoblastoma
D   hilus cell tumour
E   fibroma

Your answers: A.......B........C.......D.......E.......

26   Dyskaryotic squamous cells in a cervical smear

A   indicate dysplasia of the cervix
B   do not require follow-up or further investigation
C   can be disregarded if reported as mild (superficial cell type)
D   if severe (parabasal cell type) are an indication for further investigation by colposcopy and biopsy
E   if severe (parabasal cell type) are an indication for follow-up by cervical cytology only

Your answers: A.......B........C.......D.......E.......

27   The following tumours are hormone dependent:

A   breast carcinoma
B   squamous cell carcinoma of the cervix
C   prostatic carcinoma
D   osteosarcoma
E   colonic carcinoma

Your answers: A.......B........C.......D.......E.......

28   The following tumours are of embryonic origin:

A   dermoid cyst
B   nephroblastoma
C   glioblastoma
D   reticulum cell sarcoma
E   retinoblastoma

Your answers: A.......B........C.......D.......E.......

29   The following features are characteristic of malignant tumours:

A   the presence of metastatic growth
B   absence of mitotic figures
C   invasion of surrounding tissues
D   loss of differentiation
E   in the majority, a rapid rate of growth

Your answers: A.......B.......C.......D.......E.......

30   The following diseases produce a tuberculoid reaction:

A   sarcoidosis
B   Crohn's disease
C   primary syphilis
D   rheumatoid disease
E   hyperthyroidism

Your answers: A.......B.......C.......D.......E.......

31   The following are absolute end arteries and have no collateral circulation:

A   retinal
B   renal
C   uterine
D   splenic
E   carotid

Your answers: A.......B.......C.......D.......E.......

32   The phaeochromocytoma

A   is a tumour of adrenal medullary tissue
B   is benign in the majority of cases
C   has its maximum incidence after the menopause
D   can be associated with severe episodes of hypotension
E   is always found in the adrenal gland

Your answers: A.......B.......C.......D.......E.......

33 The human Fallopian tube

A   contains only ciliated cells
B   has four muscular layers
C   usually contains the fertilised ovum for six days
D   epithelium has cyclic variation
E   isthmo-ampullary junction is not clearly demarcated

Your answers: A.......B.......C.......D.......E.......

34 In the labia majora

A   the blood supply is derived from the internal and external pudendal arteries
B   a persistent processus vaginalis may be present
C   venous drainage does not connect with the dorsal veins of the clitoris
D   Meissner corpuscles are present
E   lymphatic systems are separate on each side

Your answers: A.......B.......C.......D.......E.......

35 The ureter

A   is lined with columnar epithelium
B   has four muscle layers
C   passes down on the psoas muscle and crosses the bifurcation of the common iliac artery
D   derives its blood supply for the upper portion from the vesical artery
E   is of mesodermal origin

Your answers: A.......B.......C.......D.......E.......

36 The bladder

A   receives parasympathetic nerve supply from S2, S3, S4
B   is lined with transitional epithelium
C   has a mobile trigone
D   muscle and mucosal walls are pierced obliquely by the ureters
E   epithelium is ectodermal in origin

Your answers: A.......B.......C.......D.......E.......

37   **The following statements relating to the ischial spines are correct:**

A   they lie between the greater and lesser sciatic notches
B   they mark the beginning of the forward curve of the birth canal
C   they are of particular prominence in the normal female pelvis
D   when the widest diameter of the fetal skull is at the level of the spines, the head is not yet engaged
E   the internal pudendal nerve lies in close relationship to the spines

Your answers: A.......B.......C.......D.......E.......

38   **The right ovary**

A   has a blood supply from the abdominal aorta
B   is attached to the anterior (inferior) layer of the broad ligament
C   has the ovarian ligament attached to its lateral pole
D   is covered by peritoneum in the adult
E   is drained by veins which go to the inferior vena cava

Your answers: A.......B.......C.......D.......E.......

39   **The uterine artery**

A   is a branch of the internal iliac artery
B   passes below the ureter in the broad ligament
C   does not supply the cervix
D   eventually forms an anastomosis with the tubal branch of the ovarian artery
E   directly supplies the round ligament

Your answers: A.......B.......C.......D.......E.......

40   **Branches of the internal iliac artery include**

A   internal pudendal
B   obturator
C   superior gluteal
D   middle rectal
E   ovarian

Your answers: A.......B.......C.......D.......E.......

41 The pudendal nerve

A   arises from sacral nerves S2, S3, S4
B   lies lateral to the pudendal vessels
C   lies medial to the ischial spine
D   passes through the greater sciatic foramen
E   terminates as the perineal nerve

Your answers: A.......B.......C.......D.......E.......

42 The femoral nerve

A   is derived from the posterior divisions of lumbar nerves 2, 3 and 4
B   lies in the iliac fossa between psoas and iliacus muscles
C   lies medial to the femoral artery
D   lies lateral to the femoral vein
E   enters the thigh inside the femoral sheath

Your answers: A.......B.......C.......D.......E.......

43 The following statements relating to the inguinal canal are correct:

A   it contains the round ligament
B   the anterior wall is mainly composed of the external oblique aponeurosis
C   the posterior wall is formed by the internal oblique muscle
D   the deep inguinal ring is superior to the inguinal ligament
E   the superficial inguinal ring has a long bony base (the pubic crest)

Your answers: A.......B.......C.......D.......E.......

44 In the healthy neonate

A   the onset of physiological jaundice is between the 6th and 8th day
B   the bowel is sterile at birth
C   urine is not normally passed until 24 hours after birth
D   the respiratory rate is in the region of 25-35 per minute
E   the ductus arteriosus closes functionally within an hour of birth

Your answers: A.......B.......C.......D.......E.......

45   The pituitary gland

A   lies superior to the sphenoid bone
B   is all ectodermal
C   has the optic chiasma anteriorly
D   is supplied from the internal carotid artery
E   lies inferior to the cavernous sinus

Your answers: A.......B.......C.......D.......E.......

46   Herpes virus hominis infection

A   in the female genital tract is predominantly of the type 3 variety
B   is usually asymptomatic
C   transmits transplacentally
D   may be transmitted to the fetus during the second stage of labour
E   occurs with lower incidence in the non-pregnant population

Your answers: A.......B.......C.......D.......E.......

47   *Clostridia* organisms

A   are primarily saprophytic
B   are aerobic
C   undergo spore formation
D   produce endotoxins
E   are typically Gram-negative

Your answers: A.......B.......C.......D.......E.......

48   *Treponema pallidum*

A   can be identified by direct light microscopy
B   can be cultured on a laboratory medium
C   is easily distinguished morphologically from *Treponema pertenue*
D   does not cause a true infection in any animal except man
E   crosses the human placenta

Your answers: A.......B.......C.......D.......E.......

49   Streptococci

A   are all Gram-positive
B   are solely aerobic
C   are the main cause of infective endocarditis
D   are arranged in characteristic grape-like clusters in Gram stained preparation
E   typically produce the enzyme coagulase

Your answers: A.......B.......C.......D.......E.......

50   The maternal serum alpha-fetoprotein concentration in pregnancy may be elevated in association with the following fetal conditions:

A   intrauterine death
B   congenital heart disease
C   twins
D   congenital nephrosis
E   microcephaly

Your answers: A.......B.......C.......D.......E.......

51   Rhesus isoimmunisation

A   is less common in ABO incompatible pregnancies
B   occurs in only 5% of exposed Rh-ve mothers
C   is usually due to anti-E
D   is due to cell bound antibodies
E   is determined by antigens limited to the red cell surface

Your answers: A.......B.......C.......D.......E.......

52   In development of the human gonads and ducts

A   differentiation occurs later in the female
B   the caudal part of the female Mullerian duct degenerates to form Gartner's duct
C   Sertoli cells are derivatives of primordial sex cells
D   the Mullerian duct is an invagination of ectodermal tissue
E   the Mullerian tubercle is the site of the future hymen

Your answers: A.......B.......C.......D.......E.......

53 **The following statements concerning autosomal recessive disorders are correct:**

A   both sexes are affected
B   the disorder is inherited from only one parent
C   the sibling of an affected child has a one in four chance of being affected
D   the rarer a recessive disease the greater the frequency of consanguinity among parents of an affected child
E   a grandparent of an affected child may be affected

Your answers: A.......B.......C.......D.......E.......

54 **The standard deviation of a group of observations**

A   is the square of the variance of the group
B   is a measure of the scatter of observations around the mean
C   has a normal Gaussian distribution
D   may be used as a basis of the calculation of x^2
E   either side of the mean encompasses 75% of the observations

Your answers: A.......B.......C.......D.......E.......

55 **In the human heart**

A   the intrinsic rate is 110/min
B   the sympathetic nervous system is predominant
C   the rate is slowed by mesenteric traction
D   the sino-atrial node is the pacemaker
E   distension of the left ventricle wall causes tachycardia

Your answers: A.......B.......C.......D.......E.......

56 **During adolescence**

A   the first evidence of sexual maturation in girls is the development of axillary hair
B   boys achieve puberty earlier than girls
C   oestrogen treatment accelerates the rate of skeletal maturation
D   mean maximum height velocity is 13 cm/year
E   the cervix remains double the length of the uterus

Your answers: A.......B.......C.......D.......E.......

57 The adult human haemoglobin A

A   has a molecular weight of 20,000
B   has a globulin portion containing predominantly alpha and gamma chains
C   has a higher affinity for oxygen than fetal haemoglobin (HgbF)
D   is produced at a rate of 6 gm. per day in normal conditions
E   contains haem groups which are porphyrin-only structures
Your answers: A.......B.......C.......D.......E.......

58 Ergometrine

A   takes 2.5 mins. to cause uterine contraction in the post-partum woman when given intramuscularly
B   has anti-emetic properties
C   may cause tachycardia
D   should be used only with caution in pre-eclamptic patients
E   is more effective towards term than in early pregnancy
Your answers: A.......B.......C.......D.......E.......

59 In the fetus

A   the umbilical arteries carry oxygenated blood
B   the ductus venosus short circuits the capillaries of the liver
C   the right atrium contains a mixture of oxygenated and venous blood
D   the foramen ovale connects the ventricles of the heart
E   the ductus arteriosus joins the aorta proximal to the aortic arch
Your answers: A.......B.......C.......D.......E.......

60 Trisomy

A   is the presence of three different cell lines in an individual
B   in all its forms can be detected by examination of the buccal smear
C   occurs with increasing frequency as maternal age increases
D   of chromosome 21 is the commonest trisomy found in live births
E   is caused by rubella infection in early pregnancy
Your answers: A.......B.......C.......D.......E.......

END OF EXAM 2

Go over your answers until the time is up. Then mark your answers according to the correct solutions given on page 89.

PRACTICE EXAM 3

60 Questions: time allowed 2 hours.
Indicate your answers (T or F) in the space provided.

1   **During the process of fertilisation and implantation**

A   fertilisation occurs in the outer third of the Fallopian tube
B   the haploid number of chromosomes results
C   the morula is enclosed by trophoblast
D   the morula actively moves along the oviduct
E   human chorionic gonadotrophin (HCG) is produced by the preimplantation embryo

Your answers: A.......B.......C.......D.......E.......

2   **Amniotic fluid**

A   has an acid pH
B   increases in volume after the 37th week
C   organic constituents are mainly lipoid
D   decreases in volume with intrauterine growth retardation
E   protein content decreases after the 26th week

Your answers: A.......B.......C.......D.......E.......

3   **Calcium absorption is**

A   increased in diets containing high protein
B   decreased in coeliac disease
C   increased in high phosphate diets
D   decreased by calcitonin
E   decreased in chronic pancreatitis

Your answers: A.......B.......C.......D.......E.......

4   **During the normal menstrual cycle in the human**

A   basal vacuolation is the earliest histological evidence of ovulation
B   gland mitosis occurs in the menstruating endometrium
C   endometrial regeneration occurs from the zona compacta
D   the secretory or postovulatory changes in the endometrium are brought about by oestrogen action
E   spiral arterial changes initiate endometrial menstrual breakdown

Your answers: A.......B.......C.......D.......E.......

31

5   Pregnancy is associated with

A   an increase in cardiac output
B   a decrease in central venous pressure
C   an increase in peripheral resistance
D   an increase in pulse rate
E   a decrease in stroke volume

Your answers: A.......B.......C.......D.......E.......

6   Respiratory changes in pregnancy include

A   increase in the total lung capacity
B   increase in the airways resistance
C   decreased subcostal angle
D   decrease in vital capacity
E   increase in the minute volume

Your answers: A.......B.......C.......D.......E.......

7   Fibrinogen

A   is synthesised in bone marrow
B   decreases in concentration during pregnancy
C   has a normal plasma concentration of 50-100 mg per 100 ml
D   is converted to fibrin by thrombin
E   synthesis is dependent on vitamin K

Your answers: A.......B.......C.......D.......E.......

8   The following statements are correct:

A   the ordinary diet in Great Britain provides 10-11 mg of iron
     each day
B   all of the daily ingested iron is absorbed
C   ingested iron is absorbed in the ferric form
D   iron is absorbed in the upper part of the jejunum and
     duodenum
E   absorbed iron combines with apoferritin in the intestinal cells
     to form ferritin

Your answers: A.......B.......C.......D.......E.......

9   Aldosterone causes

A   a fall in urinary sodium excretion
B   weight gain
C   a fall in serum chloride levels
D   increased extracellular fluid volume
E   increased potassium excretion

Your answers: A.......B.......C.......D.......E.......

10   In fat absorption and metabolism

A   dietary fat is absorbed in the stomach
B   dietary fat is absorbed in the form of chylomicrons
C   the rate of cholesterol and myelin lipid synthesis is high in
     adult central nervous tissue
D   fatty acids are a major source of oxidative energy
E   linoleic acid is an essential fatty acid

Your answers: A.......B.......C.......D.......E.......

11   During the process of glucose production and metabolism

A   the liver is the main organ of production
B   metabolism in the glycolytic pathway starts with glucose-
     6-phosphate
C   there is a net production of 4 molecules of ATP
D   the liver is the site of the gluco-regulatory action of
     glucagon
E   human growth hormone stimulates glucose uptake in fat and
     muscle

Your answers: A.......B.......C.......D.......E.......

**12   The following substances cross the placenta to the fetus against a
     concentration gradient:**

A   calcium
B   magnesium
C   amino acids
D   iron
E   fat soluble vitamins

Your answers: A.......B.......C.......D.......E.......

13 Neonatal hypocalcaemia

A   may be due to maternal dietary deficiency
B   often accompanies hypoglycaemia
C   causes permanent brain damage
D   is a common cause of convulsions
E   is seen in association with a normal maternal blood calcium concentration

Your answers: A.......B.......C.......D.......E.......

14 Prolactin

A   is produced by the anterior pituitary
B   concentration in the plasma rises in human pregnancy
C   production is increased by thyroid stimulating hormone-releasing hormone
D   plasma concentrations fall by 50% or more just before delivery in the human
E   has a long half-life in the circulation

Your answers: A.......B.......C.......D.......E.......

15 The following statements are correct:

A   thyroid stimulating hormone (TSH) is a polypeptide
B   thyroxine and tri-iodothyronine are the same
C   thyroxine stimulates oxygen consumption
D   congenital hypothyroidism (cretinism) may result from untreated maternal thyrotoxicosis (hyperthyroidism)
E   the inactive thyroid gland shows an increased amount of colloid

Your answers: A.......B.......C.......D.......E.......

16 Insulin

A   is a glycoprotein
B   is produced by the α cells
C   levels decrease and glucagon levels increase in response to hypoglycaemia
D   is not required by exercising muscle to utilise glucose
E   facilitates glycogen breakdown and increases glucose output from the liver

Your answers: A.......B.......C.......D.......E.......

17   Human chorionic gonadotrophin (HCG)

A   reaches a maximum at the end of pregnancy
B   serves as a tumour marker
C   production begins before the corpus luteum of pregnancy
D   is increased in hydatidiform mole
E   is the basis of most laboratory pregnancy tests

Your answers: A.......B.......C.......D.......E.......

18   Excess parathyroid hormone causes

A   high blood calcium
B   high blood phosphate
C   increased urinary excretion of phosphate
D   increased urinary calcium
E   increased urinary hydroxyproline excretion

Your answers: A.......B.......C.......D.......E.......

19   Oxytocin

A   is synthesised by the pituitary gland
B   rises in concentration in maternal blood before the onset of labour
C   causes milk ejection
D   is acted upon by oxytocinase
E   has biological properties overlapping with vasopressin

Your answers: A.......B.......C.......D.......E.......

20   A low level of potassium in the plasma may be caused by

A   dehydration
B   thiazide diuretics
C   acidosis
D   primary hyperaldosteronism (Conn's syndrome)
E   a beta-cell tumour of the pancreas

Your answers: A.......B.......C.......D.......E.......

21   Maternal urinary oestriol excretion

A   falls prior to abruptio placentae
B   contines to rise after term
C   is low in maternal cardiac disease
D   indicates only placental functional status
E   when falling in association with maternal hypertensive disease may indicate deteriorating fetal condition

Your answers: A.......B.......C.......D.......E.......

22   Fetal respiratory movements in utero

A   are normally present for 80% of the 24 hr period
B   occur at a frequency of 2 per minute
C   are increased in asymetrical growth retardation
D   are reduced after maternal meals
E   increase with increasing gestation

Your answers: A.......B.......C.......D.......E.......

23   Glucocorticoids

A   have their major effect on intermediary metabolism i.e. protein- carbohydrate interconversion
B   cause an increase in total body water content
C   are needed to increase liver storage of glycogen
D   have a negative feedback effect on ACTH (corticotrophin)
E   are C17 steroids

Your answers: A.......B.......C.......D.......E.......

24   The following drugs cross the placental barrier:

A   heparin
B   tetracycline
C   sulphadimidine
D   diazepam
E   salicylate

Your answers: A.......B.......C.......D.......E.......

25 Progesterone is

A   synthesised by the trophoblast
B   mainly excreted as pregnanediol glucuronide
C   synthesised from cholesterol
D   a smooth muscle stimulant
E   a glycoprotein

Your answers: A.......B.......C.......D.......E.......

26 Progestogens

A   reduce cervical mucus ferning
B   cause cessation of endometrial gland proliferation
C   increase the permeability of cervical mucus to sperms
D   are responsible for the hypertensive change in women taking combined oral contraceptives
E   inhibit uterine muscle activity

Your answers: A.......B.......C.......D.......E.......

27 Hormones from the posterior pituitary affect

A   water reabsorption in the kidney
B   uterine contractions
C   ovulation
D   milk expulsion
E   placental growth

Your answers: A.......B.......C.......D.......E.......

28 Heparin

A   crosses the placenta easily
B   remains effective many hours after stopping administration
C   prevents embolisation of an established clot
D   acts as an anti-thrombin
E   is rendered ineffective by protamine sulphate

Your answers: A.......B.......C.......D.......E.......

29   Uterine fibromyomata may undergo the following changes:

A   atrophy
B   hyaline degeneration
C   sarcomatous change
D   calcification
E   red degeneration

Your answers: A.......B.......C.......D.......E.......

30   The endometrium

A   is supplied with blood by the radial and spiral arteries
B   shows subnuclear vacuolation of the glandular epithelial cells before ovulation
C   shows tortuous lengthened glands in the secretory phase
D   shows declining glandular secretion after the 22nd day of the cycle if pregnancy fails to occur
E   divides into a superficial compact and deep spongy layer in the functional zone between the 25th and 28th day of the cycle

Your answers: A.......B.......C.......D.......E.......

31   The anterior pituitary

A   is known in part as the pars tuberalis
B   produces follicle stimulating hormone
C   lies above the optic chiasma
D   is controlled by releasing factors produced in the hypothalamus
E   produces vasopressin

Your answers: A.......B.......C.......D.......E.......

32   The following statements are correct:

A   the paramesonephric duct crosses the mesonephric duct ventrally to reach its medial side
B   the whole of the uterovaginal canal is formed by fusion of the two mesonephric ducts
C   the Mullerian tubercle is formed in the dorsal wall of the urogenital sinus
D   throughout fetal and early postnatal life the cervical portion of the uterus is larger than the body
E   the caudal part of the hindgut receives the allantois and is called the cloaca

Your answers: A.......B.......C.......D.......E.......

33 The inguinal canal

A carries the round ligament in the female
B has its posterior wall made up entirely by transversalis fascia
C is the passage between the deep and superficial rings
D may contain a congenital persistence of a peritoneal channel
E carries the ilioinguinal nerve

Your answers: A.......B.......C.......D.......E.......

34 The inguinal lymph nodes receive lymph from

A perianal skin
B the infra-umbilical region
C prostate
D testis
E clefts between the toes

Your answers: A.......B.......C.......D.......E.......

35 The following statements are correct:

A the human pronephros survives into adult life
B mesonephric vesicles give rise to the glomerulus
C the tubules, calyces, pelvis and ureter develop from the ureteric bud
D urine formation does not begin before the fifth month of fetal life
E the mature fetus may void 450 ml of urine daily into the amniotic cavity

Your answers: A.......B.......C.......D.......E.......

36 The portal and systemic venous systems anastomose at

A the rectal plexus
B the liver sinusoids
C the oesophagus
D the umbilicus
E the spleen

Your answers: A.......B.......C.......D.......E.......

37   The following conditions are X-linked:

A   congenital adrenal hyperplasia
B   Duchenne muscular dystrophy
C   classical achondroplasia
D   true hermaphroditism
E   Hurler's syndrome

Your answers: A.......B.......C.......D.......E.......

38   In Down's syndrome

A   most patients have an extra number 21 chromosome
B   trisomy is usually due to non-disjunction during meiosis
C   a female with Down's syndrome would never have a normal child
D   women over the age of 40 years have a risk of 1 in 200 of having a child with Down's syndrome
E   an affected fetus may be associated with a reduced alpha-fetoprotein concentration in amniotic fluid

Your answers: A.......B.......C.......D.......E.......

39   There is a recognisable chromosome abnormality in the following:

A   Klinefelter's syndrome
B   Tay-Sach's disease
C   achondroplasia
D   Cri du chat syndrome
E   Patau's syndrome

Your answers: A.......B.......C.......D.......E.......

40   Chromosomes

A   are usually studied after 12-24 hours culture of peripheral blood
B   are most easily identified during interphase
C   are reduced in number during the first stage of meiosis
D   are arrested in their division at anaphase to facilitate analysis in the laboratory
E   normally number 45

Your answers: A.......B.......C.......D.......E.......

41   Lymphokines

A   are antibodies arising from mast cells
B   arise from plasma cells
C   are IgE immunoglobulins
D   are responsible for immune complex formation
E   are produced by Type IV cell-mediated immune responses

Your answers: A.......B.......C.......D.......E.......

42   Human leucocyte antigens (HLA) are

A   genetically determined by the Major Histocompatibility Complex (MHC)
B   only present on leucocytes
C   usually two in number on human leucocytes
D   involved in transplantation immunity
E   glycoproteins

Your answers: A.......B.......C.......D.......E.......

43   Maternal immunoglobulins

A   never cause disease in the fetus
B   never cross the placenta
C   provide passive immunity for the newborn
D   are transferred to the baby in breast milk
E   are excreted in the urine in normal uncomplicated pregnancy

Your answers: A.......B.......C.......D.......E.......

44   Lymphocytotoxic antibodies are

A   found in all pregnant women
B   found in 10% of primigravidae
C   found in 50% of multigravidae
D   responsible for fetal abnormalities
E   associated with an increased fetal wastage

Your answers: A.......B.......C.......D.......E.......

45   The following statements are correct:

A   the mean, median and mode are the same in a normal distribution
B $P<0.05$ is more significant than $P<0.01$
C   sample standard deviation and population standard deviation are the same
D   the mode of 1,2,2,2,3,5,5,6,6,18 is 2
E   the terms prevalence and incidence are synonymous

Your answers: A.......B.......C.......D.......E.......

46   In the following diseases there is an animal reservoir of infection:

A   bubonic plague
B   diphtheria
C   anthrax
D   brucellosis
E   leptospirosis

Your answers: A.......B.......C.......D.......E.......

47   Alpha haemolytic (viridans) streptococci are commonly found to be the cause of

A   paronychia
B   subacute bacterial endocarditis
C   sore throats in children
D   acute nephritis
E   rheumatic fever

Your answers: A.......B.......C.......D.......E.......

48   Primary cytomegalovirus infection in pregnancy may cause the following in the fetus:

A   microcephaly
B   blood dyscrasias
C   myocarditis
D   pneumonia
E   enterocolitis

Your answers: A.......B.......C.......D.......E.......

49   **The following disorders can be diagnosed antenatally by analysis of amniotic fluid:**

A   phenylketonuria
B   cystic fibrosis
C   Tay-Sach's disease
D   anencephaly
E   Klinefelter's syndrome

Your answers: A.......B.......C.......D.......E.......

50   **The karyotype 47 XXY is associated with**

A   Mongolism
B   a single Barr body
C   the presence of an ovotestis
D   gynaecomastia
E   an increased incidence of mental retardation

Your answers: A.......B.......C.......D.......E.......

51   *Toxoplasma gondii*

A   is a virus
B   may be acquired by contact with cats
C   primary infection is common during pregnancy in the United Kingdom
D   maternal infection during pregnancy may cause purpura in the newborn
E   maternal infection during pregnancy may cause choroido-retinitis in the infant

Your answers: A.......B.......C.......D.......E.......

52   **Rubella infection**

A   is spread by direct contact
B   has an incubation period of 4 weeks
C   if acquired after the 16th week of pregnancy produces a congenital malformation in 30% of cases
D   the rubella specific IgM usually persists throughout pregnancy
E   may occur in subclinical forms

Your answers: A.......B.......C.......D.......E.......

53 **The vagina**

A   of the female newborn is bacteriologically sterile
B   of the neonate is colonised by Doderlein's bacilli by 72 hours of life
C   of the neonate is glycogenated
D   during adolescence demonstrates the same bacteriological flora as the vulva
E   demonstrates an acid pH until puberty

Your answers: A.......B.......C.......D.......E.......

54 *Clostridium welchii*

A   is a Gram-negative organism
B   is an aerobic organism
C   may cause post-abortal gas gangrene
D   produces a lethal exotoxin
E   is locally invasive into muscle

Your answers: A.......B.......C.......D.......E.......

55 **The following statements concerning normal flora in healthy people are correct:**

A   *Proteus* is commonly found in the bowel
B   lactobacilli are commonly found in the vagina
C   pneumococci are commonly found in the lung
D   *Streptococcus viridans* is commonly found in the mouth
E   *Escherichia coli* are commonly found in the urinary bladder

Your answers: A.......B.......C.......D.......E.......

56 **Which of the following are branches of the anterior division of the internal iliac artery:**

A   iliolumbar a.
B   internal pudendal a.
C   obturator a.
D   ovarian a.
E   superior vesical a.

Your answers: A.......B.......C.......D.......E.......

57 **The lymphatic drainage**

A   of the Fallopian tube is mainly via the para-aortic nodes
B   of the cervix includes the obturator nodes
C   of the corpus uteri includes the superficial inguinal nodes
D   of each side of the vulva do not communicate
E   of the middle third of the vagina includes the superficial inguinal nodes

Your answers: A.......B.......C.......D.......E.......

58 **The obturator nerve**

A   is formed from the posterior divisions of the 2nd, 3rd and 4th lumbar nerve roots
B   is formed within the substance of psoas major
C   supplies sensory branches to both hip and knee joints
D   has no skin distribution
E   supplies motor fibres to obturator internus

Your answers: A.......B.......C.......D.......E.......

59 **The ureter**

A   crosses superior to the uterine artery in the broad ligament
B   derives its sympathetic nerve supply from the 2nd and 3rd lumbar nerve roots
C   is widest at the pelvi-ureteric junction
D   derives its blood supply entirely from the renal and superior vesical arteries
E   cross the pelvic brim lateral to the sacroiliac joint

Your answers: A.......B.......C.......D.......E.......

60 **The ischio-rectal fossae**

A   lie inferior to the levator ani
B   lie lateral to the pudendal canal
C   have lateral walls formed in part by the obturator internus fascia
D   allow dilatation of the anal canal during defaecation
E   are separated from each other by the vagina

Your answers: A.......B.......C.......D.......E.......

END OF EXAM 3
Go over your answers until the time is up. Then mark your answers according to the correct solutions given on page 104.

PRACTICE EXAM 4

60 Questions: time allowed 2 hours.
Indicate your answers in the space provided.

1   In the lower limb

A   gluteus maximus is supplied by the superior gluteal nerve
B   piriformis inserts into the lesser trochanter of the femur
C   psoas major rotates the femur laterally
D   psoas minor is inserted into the pectineal line
E   iliacus rotates the femur medially

Your answers: A.......B.......C.......D.......E.......

2   In the anterior abdominal wall

A   the rectus abdominis lies posterior to the transversalis aponeurosis below the umbilicus
B   the external oblique muscle orginates from the lower eight ribs
C   the superior epigastric artery lies superficial to the rectus abdominis
D   the pyramidalis muscle is often absent
E   the median umbilical ligament lies deep to rectus abdominis

Your answers: A.......B.......C.......D.......E.......

3   The uterus

A   derives its nerve supply from the superior hypogastric plexus
B   derives most of its support from the broad ligaments
C   is retroverted in 15% of women
D   is completely covered with peritoneum posteriorly
E   develops from the paramesonephric duct

Your answers: A.......B.......C.......D.......E.......

4   Meckel's diverticulum

A   is present in 10% of individuals
B   lies 60-70 cm from the caecum
C   arises from the jejunum
D   may contain gastric mucosa
E   may communicate with the umbilicus

Your answers: A.......B.......C.......D.......E.......

46

5   The vagina

A   is lined by columnar epithelium
B   is kept moist mainly by secretions from Bartholin's glands
C   has its upper end above the pelvic floor
D   is surrounded by bulbospongiosus muscle at its introitus
E   has lateral walls lying in contact with each other when collapsed

Your answers: A.......B.......C.......D.......E.......

6   The femoral sheath

A   envelopes the femoral nerve
B   envelopes the femoral artery
C   lies medial to the lacunar ligament
D   is pierced by the genito-femoral nerve
E   is narrowest at its proximal end

Your answers: A.......B.......C.......D.......E.......

7   In the female urethra

A   the distal end is lined by stratified squamous epithelium
B   the intramural smooth muscle consists almost entirely of longitudinal fibres
C   is 6-7 cm long
D   the intrinsic striated muscle is thicker posteriorly
E   the sphincter urethrae is supplied by the genital branch of the genito- femoral nerve

Your answers: A.......B.......C.......D.......E.......

8   The following statements concerning the anal sphincters are correct:

A   the internal sphincter surrounds the upper 2/3 of the anal canal
B   the external sphincter surrounds the lower 2/3 of the anal canal
C   the external sphincter consists of 2 distinct muscular rings
D   the internal sphincter can maintain continence of faeces and flatus acting alone
E   the internal sphincter is innervated by the inferior hypogastric plexus

Your answers: A.......B.......C.......D.......E.......

9   **The following statements concerning the lumbar and sacral nerves are correct:**

A   the ilio-inguinal nerve arises from the 2nd lumbar nerve root

B   the genito-femoral nerve arises from the 1st and 2nd lumbar nerve roots

C   the lateral cutaneous nerve of the thigh arises from the anterior divisions of the 2nd and 3rd lumbar nerve roots

D   the pudendal nerve arises from the posterior divisions of the 2nd, 3rd, and 4th sacral nerve roots

E   the perineal branch of S4 supplies the skin of the anal margin

Your answers: A.......B.......C.......D.......E.......

10   **Insulin administration leads to**

A   a fall in serum potassium
B   nucleic acid synthesis
C   gluconeogenesis
D   lipogenesis
E   esterification of fatty acids

Your answers: A.......B.......C.......D.......E.......

11   **The anterior pituitary**

A   develops as a diverticulum from the floor of the diencephalon
B   contains no nerve elements
C   receives blood supply from the internal carotid arteries
D   produces FSH within its basophil cells
E   produces oxytocin within acidophil cells

Your answers: A.......B.......C.......D.......E.......

12   **Cortisol**

A   enhances gluconeogenesis
B   reduces fibrous tissue formation
C   decreases gastric acid production
D   decreases the inflammatory response
E   lowers eosinophil count

Your answers: A.......B.......C.......D.......E.......

13   Cortisol binding

A   is increased in pregnancy
B   is increased following oestrogen administration
C   is increased in cirrhosis
D   is increased in some dysproteinaemias
E   is mainly to α-globulin

Your answers: A.......B.......C.......D.......E.......

14   In the human, fertilisation normally occurs

A   in the ampullary region of the Fallopian tube
B   after extrusion of the first polar body
C   within 48 hours of ovulation
D   14 days before implantation
E   in the presence of cervical mucus ferning

Your answers: A.......B.......C.......D.......E.......

15   Ovulation occurs

A   before the biphasic rise in temperature
B   before the LH (luteinizing hormone) surge
C   following follicular ripening by FSH (follicle stimulating hormone)
D   infrequently in women with amenorrhoea
E   after the disappearance of cervical mucus ferning

Your answers: A.......B.......C.......D.......E.......

16   The plasma concentrations of the following coagulation factors increase in normal pregnancy:

A   I-fibrinogen
B   X-Stuart-Prower factor
C   VII-proconvertin
D   VIII-antihaemophilic globulin
E   XI-plasma thromboplastin antecedent

Your answers: A.......B.......C.......D.......E.......

17   Trophoblast

A   enters the maternal circulation in normal pregnancy
B   is lysed in the maternal lung
C   is genetically maternal
D   produces human chorionic gonadotrophins
E   is immunologically inert

Your answers: A.......B.......C.......D.......E.......

18   Fetal pulmonary maturity

A   is delayed in diabetic pregnancies
B   normally occurs before the 36th week of gestation
C   is influenced by corticosteroid levels
D   is controlled by α-fetoprotein
E   is delayed in intra-uterine growth retardation

Your answers: A.......B.......C.......D.......E.......

19   The increased uterine blood flow in pregnancy is contributed to by

A   an increase in the number of uterine arterioles
B   increased diameter of placental blood vessels
C   reduced vascular resistance in the uterus
D   increased angiotensin II levels
E   increased blood volume

Your answers: A.......B.......C.......D.......E.......

20   Human chorionic gonadotrophin

A   is produced by the trophoblast
B   is produced by fetal liver
C   may be immunosuppressive
D   reaches a peak in the second trimester of pregnancy
E   is produced by some non-trophoblastic tumours

Your answers: A.......B.......C.......D.......E.......

21   In renal function

A   glomerular filtration can be measured using inulin
B   changes in osmotic pressure can cause significant changes in glomerular filtration
C   carbonic anhydrase increases the rate of conversion of H_2CO_3 into H^+ and HCO_3^-
D   90% of filtered water is reabsorbed
E   the ascending loop of Henle is relatively impermeable to water

Your answers: A.......B.......C.......D.......E.......

22   The following are therapeutically radiosensitive human genital tract tumours:

A   squamous cell carcinoma of cervix
B   adenocarcinoma of cervix
C   carcinoma of vulva
D   dysgerminoma
E   adenocarcinoma of endometrium

Your answers: A.......B.......C.......D.......E.......

23   Hypokalaemia causes

A   paralytic ileus
B   mental confusion
C   increased sensitivity of the renal tubules to antidiuretic hormone (ADH)
D   aciduria
E   elevation of the ST segment on the electrocardiogram

Your answers: A.......B.......C.......D.......E.......

24   The following are carcinogenic:

A   formaldehyde
B   asbestos
C   chromium
D   nickel
E   wood dust

Your answers: A.......B.......C.......D.......E.......

25   The following statements about the pathology of degeneration are correct:

A   in hydropic degeneration the cytoplasm has a granular appearance
B   in hyaline degeneration the cytoplasm is basophilic
C   pyknosis refers to fragmentation of nuclear material
D   karyorrhexis refers to clumping of nuclear material
E   striated muscle may undergo necrosis during acute fevers

Your answers: A.......B.......C.......D.......E.......

26   Cofactors, prosthetic groups and metal activators

A   are essential for certain enzyme reactions
B   can be closely related chemically to one another
C   are irreversibly altered at the end of a reaction
D   arise from dietary sources
E   function in the same way as the enzyme substrate

Your answers: A.......B.......C.......D.......E.......

27   Squamous metaplasia may occur in the following sites:

A   cervix uteri
B   gall bladder
C   liver
D   stomach
E   bronchus

Your answers: A.......B.......C.......D.......E.......

28   In obstructive jaundice

A   plasma levels of conjugated bilirubin are normal
B   there is an increased amount of stercobilinogen in the faeces
C   there is an increased amount of urobilinogen in the urine
D   bilirubin is present in the urine
E   there is increased hepatic production of alkaline phosphatase

Your answers: A.......B.......C.......D.......E.......

29   Histological features of sarcoidosis include

A   epithelioid cells
B   caseation
C   round cell infiltration
D   Langhan's giant cells
E   Schaumann bodies

Your answers: A.......B.......C.......D.......E.......

30   Features of benign tumours usually include

A   an intact capsule
B   local invasion
C   well differentiated cell types
D   pleomorphism
E   regional lymphadenopathy

Your answers: A.......B.......C.......D.......E.......

31   Squamous metaplasia

A   is a form of carcinoma in situ
B   may follow malignant change
C   occurs in the bladder
D   occurs in the uterus
E   is the same as anaplasia

Your answers: A.......B.......C.......D.......E.......

32   The following statements about maternal and fetal thyroid function are correct:

A   the fetal thyroid traps iodine from the 6th week of gestation onwards
B   the fetal pituitary starts to secrete TSH in the second trimester
C   maternal TSH freely crosses the placental barrier
D   cretins have high TSH levels in the first week of life
E   levels of free thyroxine are lower in pregnancy than in a non-pregnant adult

Your answers: A.......B.......C.......D.......E.......

33   Human placental lactogen

A   increases insulin resistance
B   promotes fat mobilisation
C   cannot be detected in maternal serum until the 14th week of pregnancy
D   shows an elevated level in twin pregnancy
E   shows a normal level in trophoblastic disease

Your answers: A.......B.......C.......D.......E.......

34   Cyproterone acetate

A   decreases gonadotrophin secretion
B   is used to induce ovulation
C   is used in the treatment of virilism
D   is safe in pregnant patients
E   exhibits strong progestogenic activity when acetylated

Your answers: A.......B.......C.......D.......E.......

35   Raised serum levels of follicle stimulating hormone are found in

A   association with combined oestrogen/progesterone contraceptive use
B   post-menopausal women
C   Sheehan's syndrome
D   Turner's syndrome
E   pure gonadal dysgenesis

Your answers: A.......B.......C.......D.......E.......

36   Cortisol

A   is produced by the zona glomerulosa of the adrenal cortex
B   has a diurnal rhythm with its lowest level present in the morning
C   is excreted in the urine as a 17 oxogenic steroid
D   production is increased by hypoglycaemia
E   when produced in excess is associated with generalised obesity

Your answers: A.......B.......C.......D.......E.......

37 **The following statements concerning adrenal metabolism are correct:**

A   primary hyperaldosteronism (Conn's syndrome) leads to high plasma potassium levels

B   ACTH acts by entering cells and increasing enzyme production

C   renin acts on the juxtaglomerular apparatus to produce angiotensin I

D   ACTH is necessary for the production of aldosterone

E   sodium depletion stimulates renin release

Your answers: A.......B.......C.......D.......E.......

38 **Increased capillary permeability in acute inflammation is produced by**

A   histamine

B   bradykinin

C   angiotensin

D   5 hydroxytryptamine

E   prostacyclin

Your answers: A.......B.......C.......D.......E.......

39 **Cephaloridine**

A   can be given orally

B   is hepatotoxic

C   is more toxic when given in combination with frusemide

D   contains a β-lactam ring

E   may cause anaphylaxis in patients who are allergic to penicillin

Your answers: A.......B.......C.......D.......E.......

40 **Beta-blocking drugs**

A   may cause hypoglycaemia in the neonate

B   improve asthma

C   are contraindicated in heart block

D   lower blood pressure by reducing peripheral vascular resistance

E   are used in the treatment of thyrotoxicosis

Your answers: A.......B.......C.......D.......E.......

41   Hydrocortisone

A   causes eosinophilia
B   increases urinary calcium excretion
C   causes negative nitrogen balance
D   decreases urinary potassium excretion
E   decreases gluconeogenesis

Your answers: A.......B.......C.......D.......E.......

42   Bromocriptine

A   is a derivative of ergot
B   is a vasoconstrictor
C   inhibits prolactin secretion at the pituitary level
D   is teratogenic
E   causes raised prolactin levels to return to normal after 48-72 hours of treatment

Your answers: A.......B.......C.......D.......E.......

43   In sex steroid metabolism

A   androstenedione is the main androgen
B   the normal ranges of testosterone in the male and female overlap
C   in women more than 50% of circulating testosterone is secreted by the adrenals
D   in women more than 50% of circulating dehydro-epiandrosterone is ovarian in origin
E   testosterone and androstenedione are readily inter-convertible

Your answers: A.......B.......C.......D.......E.......

44   Passive immunisation is used in the prophylaxis of the following conditions:

A   actinomycosis
B   pertussis
C   rubella in pregnancy
D   syphilis
E   tuberculosis

Your answers: A.......B.......C.......D.......E.......

45   A toxoid is a toxin which has been treated so that it

A   can no longer be phagocytosed
B   it can no longer stimulate an immune response
C   is still antigenic but not toxic
D   is still toxic but not antigenic
E   no longer gives a precipitin reaction with antibody

Your answers: A.......B.......C......D.......E.......

46   Bacteraemic shock

A   is caused by an exotoxin
B   may be associated with leukopoenia
C   is usually caused by staphylococci
D   is improved by massive doses of steroids
E   is associated with sympathetic nervous activation

Your answers: A.......B.......C......D.......E.......

47   The following maternal infections cause congenital infection in the neonate

A   coxsackie B virus
B   cytomegalovirus
C   hepatitis B
D   poliomyelitis
E   herpes simplex (type 2)

Your answers: A.......B.......C......D.......E.......

48   Vitamin C is

A   found only in animal foodstuffs
B   necessary for wound healing
C   fat soluble
D   rapidly destroyed by heating
E   preserved by food freezing

Your answers: A.......B.......C......D.......E.......

49   The tricarboxylic (Krebs) cycle

A   is a source of adenosine triphosphate (ATP)
B   has a purely catabolic function
C   converts metabolic energy into chemical energy
D   provides for the complete combustion of fatty acids
E   requires co-enzyme for its continued operation

Your answers: A.......B.......C.......D.......E.......

50   Vitamin B$_{12}$

A   requires intrinsic factor for absorption
B   is water soluble
C   deficiency can be treated by oral supplementation
D   is only obtained from animal sources in the diet
E   is destroyed by cooking

Your answers: A.......B.......C.......D.......E.......

51   The normal 'herniation' of abdominal contents through the fetal abdominal wall

A   occurs during the 11th to 14th week of gestation
B   contains the fetal stomach
C   undergoes rotation in a clockwise direction
D   is supplied by the coeliac artery
E   is attached to the allantois at its apex

Your answers: A.......B.......C.......D.......E.......

52   The Mullerian ducts

A   are derived from intermediate cell mass mesoderm
B   appear between the 8th and 9th weeks of embryonic development
C   develop lateral to the Wolffian ducts
D   fuse throughout their length by the 12th week of fetal development
E   become the sinovaginal bulbs in their lower part

Your answers: A.......B.......C.......D.......E.......

53 Alleles are

A   structural gene products
B   regulatory gene products
C   dominant genes
D   non-identical genes at the same locus
E   broken off gene fragments

Your answers: A.......B.......C.......D.......E.......

54 The T-lymphocyte population

A   is responsible for cell-mediated immune response
B   recirculates through the reticulo-endothelial system
C   populate the paracortical areas of the central lymphoid tissue
D   comprise 70% of blood lymphocytes
E   arise from stem cells in the thymus

Your answers: A.......B.......C.......D.......E.......

55 A report comparing the effectiveness of drugs X and Y states that drug X was more effective in certain respects to a significant level (p<0.01). It can be concluded that

A   the observed greater effectiveness is statistically significant
B   at least 1000 patients were studied
C   the chances of being improved by drug X are more than 99% in each case
D   side effects occurred in less than 1 in 100
E   this was a controlled randomised trial

Your answers: A.......B.......C.......D.......E.......

56 The cervix

A   undergoes cyclical changes during the menstrual cycle
B   loses its lining during menstruation
C   has columnar epithelium lining the canal
D   produces a thick scanty discharge at ovulation
E   has the same proportion of muscle in its wall as the corpus uteri

Your answers: A.......B.......C.......D.......E.......

57   The inguinal ligament

A   forms the floor of the inguinal canal
B   is inferior to the deep inguinal ring
C   is attached laterally to the anterior inferior iliac spine
D   is the lower border of the external oblique aponeurosis
E   is superior to the ilio-inguinal nerve

Your answers: A.......B.......C.......D.......E.......

58   The trigone of the bladder

A   develops from the urogenital sinus
B   lies between the ureteric orifices and the urachus
C   is more sensitive than the urethra
D   is the least mobile part of the bladder
E   is always smooth

Your answers: A.......B.......C.......D.......E.......

59   The typical female bony pelvis

A   has a transverse diameter at the inlet greater than the antero-posterior diameter
B   has an obstetric conjugate of 11-12 cm
C   is funnel-shaped
D   has an obtuse greater sciatic notch
E   has a subpubic angle > 90 degrees

Your answers: A.......B.......C.......D.......E.......

60   The femoral canal

A   is medial to the femoral vein at the proximal end
B   contains the femoral branch of the genito-femoral nerve
C   has the femoral ring at its lower end
D   contains lymph vessels
E   is posterior to the inguinal ligament at its proximal end

Your answers: A.......B.......C.......D.......E.......

END OF EXAM 4

Go over your answers until the time is up. Then mark your answers according to the correct solutions given on page 120.

PRACTICE EXAM 5

60 Questions: time allowed 2 hours.
Indicate your answers (T or F) in the space provided.

1   The right ovary

A   receives its blood supply from the aorta
B   is attached to the anterior leaf of the broad ligament
C   is attached to the suspensory ligament of ovary at its lateral pole
D   is covered by peritoneum in the adult
E   has veins which drain to the inferior vena cava

Your answers: A.......B.......C.......D.......E.......

2   The middle third of the vagina

A   has a stratified squamous keratinizing epithelium
B   is related to the pouch of Douglas posteriorly
C   receives part of its blood supply from the inferior vesical arteries
D   is mesodermal in origin
E   is derived from the mesonephric duct

Your answers: A.......B.......C.......D.......E.......

3   The ureter

A   is an abdominal organ in 50% of its length
B   is closely related to the infundibulo-pelvic ligament
C   receives its main blood supply directly from the aorta
D   lies on psoas major
E   is adherent to the overlying peritoneum

Your answers: A.......B.......C.......D.......E.......

4   The pudendal nerve

A   innervates the internal sphincter of the rectum
B   is sensory to the skin of the labia
C   runs in the roof of the ischio-rectal fossa
D   arises from the same nerve roots as the nerve to the obturator internus muscle
E   is formed at the lower part of the greater sciatic foramen

Your answers: A.......B.......C.......D.......E.......

61

5   The Fallopian tube

A   is lined by ciliated columnar epithelium
B   is attached by the fimbria to the lateral pole of the ovary
C   undergoes cyclical changes during the menstrual cycle
D   arises from the paramesonephric duct
E   is narrower at its lateral than medial end

Your answers: A.......B.......C.......D.......E.......

6   The uterus

A   gets its entire blood supply from the uterine arteries
B   is kept in position mainly by the round ligaments
C   has as much fibrous tissue as muscle in its wall
D   has no sympathetic nerve activity
E   has an isthmus only after 12 weeks gestation

Your answers: A.......B.......C.......D.......E.......

7   The broad ligament

A   contains tissues of mesonephric origin
B   has the Fallopian tube in its upper free border
C   has the ovarian artery in its lower attached border
D   has the ureter passing forwards in its lower attached border
E   has the ovarian ligament in its posterior fold

Your answers: A.......B.......C.......D.......E.......

8   The levator ani

A   consists of smooth muscle
B   plays a part in maintaining the position of the uterus
C   is supplied by nerves from the lumbar plexus
D   has no sphincteric action in relation to the anal canal
E   is attached to the pelvic bones

Your answers: A.......B.......C.......D.......E.......

9   The female breast

A   is developmentally a collection of modified sweat glands
B   is drained mainly by lymphatics going direct to the supraclavicular nodes
C   develops a large amount of secretory tissue at puberty
D   has a separate duct for each lobe, opening onto the nipple
E   never extends laterally over serratus anterior

Your answers: A.......B.......C.......D.......E.......

10   Cardiac output

A   need not increase when the heart rate increases and is irregular
B   increases when the subject changes from the standing to the supine position
C   is commonly expressed as the combined outputs of both ventricles per minute
D   is increased reflexly in a hot climate
E   is the product of heart rate and stroke volume

Your answers: A.......B.......C.......D.......E.......

11   A sustained arterial hypertension may be due to

A   excessive aldosterone secretion
B   left ventricular hypertrophy
C   excessive secretion of adrenocorticotrophic hormone
D   hypoxia consequent to chronic respiratory failure
E   drug therapy with methyl dopa

Your answers: A.......B.......C.......D.......E.......

12   Total cerebral blood flow is most markedly increased by

A   hypercapnia
B   hypoxia
C   cerebral activity
D   vasomotor reflexes
E   increase in mean arterial pressure

Your answers: A.......B.......C.......D.......E.......

13   Carbon dioxide is transported in the blood

A   in combination with haemoglobin
B   as hydrochloric acid
C   in combination with plasma proteins
D   mainly as bicarbonate
E   in physical solution in plasma

Your answers: A.......B.......C.......D.......E.......

14   The respiratory centre

A   is situated in the medulla oblongata
B   is inhibited during vomiting
C   sends out regular impulses to the inspiratory muscles during
     quiet respiration
D   is reflexly regulated by vagal impulses
E   is sensitive to blood pH alterations

Your answers: A.......B.......C.......D.......E.......

15   The following substances are essential for erythrocyte production:

A   iron
B   folic acid
C   nicotinic acid
D   vitamin B_{12}
E   myoglobin

Your answers: A.......B.......C.......D.......E.......

16   Renal blood flow is

A   reduced during fear and emotional stress
B   unchanged by noradrenaline administration
C   greater per unit mass of tissue in the medulla than in the
     cortex
D   determined by the metabolic needs of the kidney
E   reduced when arterial pressure falls, by about the same
     percentage

Your answers: A.......B.......C.......D.......E.......

17   Glomerular filtration rate may be measured by

A   inulin
B   insulin
C   para-aminohippuric acid
D   glucagon
E   glucose

Your answers: A.......B.......C.......D.......E.......

18   Normal micturition

A   depends on the integrity of a sacral spinal reflex arc
B   is prevented by sectioning the sensory nerves supplying the bladder
C   may occur with spinal transection in the thoracic region
D   follows activation of the sympathetic nerves to the bladder
E   is under voluntary control in healthy young adults

Your answers: A.......B.......C.......D.......E.......

19   Severe diarrhoea could result in

A   hypokalaemia
B   hypernatraemia
C   death
D   shock
E   increased peripheral resistance

Your answers: A.......B.......C.......D.......E.......

20   The following changes occur during normal pregnancy:

A   blood pressure tends to be elevated in the second trimester
B   cardiac output rises only during the second and third trimesters
C   heart rate rises by 20%
D   plasma volume rises by 40%
E   stroke volume is unchanged

Your answers: A.......B.......C.......D.......E.......

21   Factors necessary for blood coagulation include

A   fibrinogen
B   prothrombin
C   Christmas factor
D   heparin
E   calcium

Your answers: A.......B.......C.......D.......E.......

22   The following are not cardinal signs of acute inflammation:

A   heat
B   pain
C   swelling
D   fever
E   turgidity of the tissues

Your answers: A.......B.......C.......D.......E.......

23   The following are chemical mediators of inflammation:

A   5-hydroxytryptamine
B   bradykinin
C   proconvertin
D   prostaglandin
E   kallikrein

Your answers: A.......B.......C.......D.......E.......

24   Macrophages

A   are derived from blood monocytes
B   are phagocytic
C   produce cellular antibodies
D   play an essential role in coagulation
E   can fuse to form giant cells

Your answers: A.......B.......C.......D.......E.......

25   The main hormones secreted by the adrenal cortex

A   include cortisol, corticosterone, dehydroepiandrosterone, cholesterol and aldosterone
B   are excreted mainly in the bile after conjugation in the liver
C   are divided functionally into mineralo - corticoids, gluco-corticoids and sex hormones
D   are largely bound to plasma proteins
E   are all solely under the control of ACTH

Your answers: A.......B.......C.......D.......E.......

26   A typical tuberculous follicle contains

A   a central mass of caseation
B   epithelioid cells
C   polymorphonuclear cells
D   giant cells
E   fibrous tissue

Your answers: A.......B.......C.......D.......E.......

27   Teratomas commonly arise in

A   ovary
B   heart
C   testis
D   mediastinum
E   sacrum

Your answers: A.......B.......C.......D.......E.......

28   The following tumours are benign:

A   papilloma
B   seminoma
C   fibroma
D   multiple myeloma
E   neurofibroma

Your answers: A.......B.......C.......D.......E.......

29   The following tumours arise in the ovary:

A   nephroblastoma
B   cystadenoma
C   granulosa cell tumour
D   neuroblastoma
E   teratoma

Your answers: A.......B.......C.......D.......E.......

30   The common primary urinary tract calculi are composed of

A   urate
B   bile
C   oxalate
D   cholesterol
E   silica

Your answers: A.......B.......C.......D.......E.......

31   The following may be constituents of emboli:

A   clot
B   tumour
C   fat
D   calculi
E   gas

Your answers: A.......B.......C.......D.......E.......

32   Aldosterone

A   is secreted by cells of the zona glomerulosa
B   production is increased by a fall in plasma renin
C   production is increased by a decrease in plasma osmolality
D   levels rise in normal pregnancy
E   is secreted in response to hyperkalaemia

Your answers: A.......B.......C.......D.......E.......

33   Parathormone

A   is produced by the C-cells of the thyroid gland
B   decreases urinary excretion of calcium
C   level in the blood increases when serum calcium falls
D   depresses activity of the anterior pituitary
E   is independent of magnesium levels

Your answers: A.......B.......C.......D.......E.....

34   Prostaglandins

A   are involved in the aetiology of excessive menstrual loss
B   have no role in the process of ovulation
C   are implicated in the onset of labour
D   cannot be manufactured effectively
E   are implicated in dysmenorrhoea

Your answers: A.......B.......C.......D.......E.......

35   The mode of action of the following cytotoxic agents is:

A   vinblastine — antimetabolite
B   tamoxifen — oestrogen agonist
C   5-fluorouracil — alkylating agent
D   adriamycin — antibiotic
E   cyclophosphamide — alkylating agent

Your answers: A.......B.......C.......D.......E.......

36   In the days following ovulation

A   the basal body temperature falls
B   the endometrium undergoes secretory changes
C   the plasma progesterone concentration falls
D   cervical mucus becomes scanty and more viscous
E   plasma luteinising hormone level falls

Your answers: A.......B.......C.......D.......E.......

37   Human chorionic gonadotrophin (HCG)

A   is a steroid
B   may be measured by radio-immuno-assay
C   acts on the uterus to maintain early pregnancy
D   production is highest in the third trimester of pregnancy
E   may provoke lutein cyst formation

Your answers: A.......B.......C.......D.......E.......

38   Spermatozoa

A   contain 23 chromosomes
B   are produced at a faster rate when testicular temperature is raised
C   require testosterone for normal development
D   require follicle stimulating hormone (FSH) for normal development
E   are produced from spermatogonia in approximately 20 days

Your answers: A.......B.......C.......D.......E.......

39   Bromocriptine

A   inhibits prolactin secretion at the pituitary level
B   may be used to suppress puerperal lactation
C   is not used to treat hyperprolactinaemic hypogonadism
D   is safe in the treatment of acromegaly
E   is a dopamine antagonist

Your answers: A.......B.......C.......D.......E.......

40   The following drugs are bacteriocidal:

A   penicillin
B   tetracycline
C   chloramphenicol
D   sulphonamide
E   streptomycin

Your answers: A.......B.......C.......D.......E.......

41 Oxytocin

A   has an antidiuretic effect
B   is produced by the anterior pituitary
C   stimulates milk formation
D   is a steroid hormone
E   has effects on the uterus which are potentiated by oestrogen

Your answers: A.......B.......C.......D.......E.......

42 Thyroxine

A   formation requires the amino acid tyrosine
B   is less than 80% bound to plasma proteins
C   is essential for skeletal development
D   increases oxygen consumption in the brain
E   leads to an increased serum cholesterol level when present in
     excess in the circulation

Your answers: A.......B.......C.......D.......E.......

43 The following drugs are teratogenic:

A   cyclophosphamide
B   penicillin
C   heparin
D   testosterone
E   sodium barbitone

Your answers: A.......B.......C.......D.......E.......

44 The following are common pathogens of the urinary tract:

A   *Escherichia coli*
B   *Proteus mirabilis*
C   *Klebsiella aerogenes*
D   *Neisseria gonorrhoea*
E   *Clostridium welchii*

Your answers: A.......B.......C.......D.......E.......

45 Candida albicans

A   is a bacterium
B   grows readily in Sabouraud's medium
C   has an increased incidence in diabetes mellitus
D   is characterised by a flagellum
E   is treated by nystatin

Your answers: A.......B.......C.......D.......E.......

46 The gonococcus

A   is a Gram-positive organism
B   grows well in anaerobic conditions
C   occasionally causes a disseminated infection
D   can cause Bartholinitis
E   is always penicillin sensitive

Your answers: A.......B.......C.......D.......E.......

47 Tuberculosis

A   of the genital tract commonly originates in the lungs
B   can cause sterility
C   does not occur in pregnant women
D   is satisfactorily treated by a 3 month course of para-amino
    salicylic acid
E   organisms resist decolourisation by 20% sulphuric acid after
    Ziehl Neelson staining

Your answers: A.......B.......C.......D.......E.......

48 In the blood in pregnancy

A   the total red cell mass increases during the second trimester
B   the plasma volume is expanded more in cases of pregnancy
    induced hypertension than normal pregnancy of the same
    gestation
C   a neutrophil leucocytosis is characteristic
D   the mean corpuscular haemoglobin concentration increases in
    folate deficiency
E   a mean red cell volume of 75 fl at 16 weeks gestation is of no
    clinical significance

Your answers: A.......B.......C.......D.......E.......

49   Plasma protein bound iodine concentrations are raised in

A   pregnancy
B   combined oestrogen/progesterone oral contraceptive users
C   nephrosis
D   salicylate users
E   androgen therapy

Your answers: A.......B.......C.......D.......E.......

50   Vitamin K

A   is required for the synthesis of prothrombin
B   is water soluble
C   deficiency may contribute to haemorrhagic disease of the newborn
D   deficiency may result from the use of broad spectrum antibiotics
E   may be deficient in the diet of certain food fadists

Your answers: A.......B.......C.......D.......E.......

51   In the development of the female genital tract

A   the Mullerian ducts fuse at their lower end to form the uterus and cervix
B   the Fallopian tubes are formed from the Wolffian ducts
C   the urogenital sinus receives the mesonephric ducts
D   the lower part of the vagina is derived from the sinovaginal bulbs
E   the urogenital sinus is continuous with the allantois

Your answers: A.......B.......C.......D.......E.......

52   Amniotic fluid

A   volume is related to gestational age
B   has no contributions from the fetal kidneys
C   alphafetoprotein level increases with gestation in the second trimester of pregnancy
D   contains no creatinine
E   osmolality increases to term

Your answers: A.......B.......C.......D.......E.......

53 **The following genetic conditions are sex-linked:**

A   the 'hairy pinna' trait
B   cleft palate
C   Hurler's syndrome (type I mucopolysaccharidosis)
D   achondroplasia
E   congenital ichthyosis

Your answers: A.......B.......C.......D.......E.......

54 **The standard deviation**

A   is a test of significance
B   is a measure of the scatter of observations about their mean
C   is only meaningful if the observations have a normal distribution
D   is calculated from the mean and number of observations alone
E   is the same as a centile

Your answers: A.......B.......C.......D.......E.......

55 **Arginine vasopressin**

A   is produced by cells of the anterior pituitary gland
B   increases the permeability of the collecting ducts of the kidney to water
C   is released in response to alcohol consumption
D   is produced in excess in diabetes insipidus
E   is a decapeptide

Your answers: A.......B.......C.......D.......E.......

56 **During respiration**

A   the amount of air that moves into the lungs with each respiration is the tidal volume
B   the volume inspired with a maximal inspiratory effort in excess of the tidal volume, is the total lung volume
C   the respiratory dead space is that space occupied by gas that does not exchange with blood in the pulmonary vessels
D   the functional residual capacity is reduced in pregnancy
E   the vital capacity is the greatest amount of air that can be expired after a passive expiration

Your answers: A.......B.......C.......D.......E.......

57   Gastrin

A   is an enzyme produced in the stomach
B   stimulates the production of acid by the stomach
C   is produced in increased amount in response to protein meals
D   is secreted by the neck cells of the gastric glands
E   effects are mimicked by histamine

Your answers: A.......B.......C.......D.......E.......

58   In relation to nerve transmission

A   acetycholine is the transmitter at all synapses between pre- and post-ganglionic fibres of the autonomic nervous system
B   noradrenaline is the transmitter at most post-ganglionic parasympathetic endings
C   5-hydroxytryptamine is a neurotransmitter
D   impulses may be transmitted in both directions across a synapse
E   synapses are less sensitive to hypoxia than nerve fibres

Your answers: A.......B.......C.......D.......E.......

59   The following structures are activated in response to acetylcholine:

A   the ciliary muscle of the eye
B   sweat glands
C   bronchial muscle
D   the gall bladder
E   the arrectores pilorum

Your answers: A.......B.......C.......D.......E.......

60   Folic acid

A   deficiency leads to megaloblastic anaemia
B   is water soluble
C   does not require gastric intrinsic factor for its absorption
D   is found only in animal foods
E   is necessary for nucleic acid synthesis

Your answers: A.......B.......C.......D.......E.......

END OF EXAM 5

Go over your answers until the time is up. Then mark your answers according to the correct solutions given on page 137.

ANSWERS AND EXPLANATIONS

ANSWERS TO PRACTICE EXAM 1
The correct answer options are given against each question.

1 A C

Prolactin is a protein of molecular weight 20,000, and structurally related to human placental lactogen. It is secreted by the acidophil cells of the anterior pituitary (along with growth hormone). A prolactin inhibitory factor is secreted by the hypothalamus and passes down the hypothalamo-hypophyseal portal system to the anterior pituitary. Therefore section of the stalk reduces this inhibitor and increases circulating prolactin levels. Chlorpromazine increases prolactin secretion probably by blocking receptors involved in the production of prolactin inhibiting hormone. It is normally measured by a radioimmunoassay technique.

2 A C D E

There is an increase in the glomerular filtration rate in normal pregnancy. This leads to an increased excretion of folate and glucose. Because of the latter the renal threshold may be reached and glycosuria may appear in pregnancy. Urate excretion increases by 40%. Ureteric dilatation is known to occur, possibly due to a progesterone effect

3 A C E

Acetylcholine has been shown to be the transmitter substance released by pre-ganglionic fibres of both sympathetic and parasympathetic systems. Post-ganglionic fibres of the parasympathetic system also secrete acetylcholine, although with a few exceptions (e.g. sweat glands) sympathetic post-ganglionic fibres have noradrenaline as their transmitter. Interneurones of sympathetic ganglia secrete dopamine. Acetylcholine is very quickly hydrolysed by a series of enzymes called cholinesterases which are present in high concentration at nerve terminals; pseudocholinesterase is present in plasma. Strychnine is a natural alkaloid, poisoning with which produces convulsions by abolishing the normal inhibitory effects of interneurones within the cord on spinal reflexes.

4 A E

The first step in the extrinsic pathway is the formation of a complex between tissue factors and factor VII. Plasmin acts on fibrinogen and fibrin, splitting them into a heterogenous mixture of small peptides known collectively as fibrin degradation products. Platelet aggregation is the primary event in coagulation in small blood vessels. Thrombasthenia is an autosomal recessive disorder resulting in a haemorrhagic tendency, the platelets failing to aggregate properly. Platelet deficiency is thrombocytopenia. Vitamin K is essential for the 8-carboxylation of specific glutamic acid residues in factors II, VII, IX and X; without it these factors do not bind calcium and do not form complexes with phospholipid.

5   B C E
During exercise, the muscles produce CO_2, but exercise produces only a slight fall in pH (by approximately 0.05) due to the buffering effect of blood and compensatory increase in the rate and depth of breathing. Stroke volume increases during severe exercise. The systolic blood pressure rises more than the diastolic blood pressure (increasing the pulse pressure) but in light exercise increased output is achieved by an increased heart rate. Body temperature rises during exercise; during the first 30-60 minutes of exercise, not all the extra heat is dissipated and temperature consequently rises. Thereafter the elevated body temperature is maintained within narrow limits.

6   A C E
The pulse rate is increased in normal healthy pregnancy. Serum colloid osmotic pressure falls by 20% due to the increase in plasma volume. Respiratory rate increases in late pregnancy leading to a 20% decrease in pCO_2. Gastric emptying time is increased in normal pregnancy.

7   D E
Peripheral resistance has fallen by approximately 40% in the second trimester of normal pregnancy. Plasma renin activity in plasma shows a considerable increase in pregnancy, up to 5-10 times the non-pregnant level. The source is thought to be the maternal kidney and not the fetus or placenta. Cardiac output increases by 30%. There is a marked increase in aldosterone production and excretion.

8   E
During physiological filling of the bladder the intravesical pressure increases minimally with intravesical urine volume; during cystometric assessment at rapid filling rates (e.g. 100 ml/min) the pressure rise should be less than 15 cm water at capacity. The first sensation of an urge to void is usually felt at around half bladder capacity, or 150-300 ml; this sensation is independent of detrusor pressure. The bladder and urethra possess both parasympathetic and sympathetic nerve supply; normal micturition is dependent upon the former but it seems that the sympathetic control is more important to the filling and storage phases than to the voiding phase of the micturition cycle. Following spinal cord transection at any level above the conus medullaris, after recovery from the phase of

spinal shock, a voiding reflex may return, although this is likely to be of dyssynergic pattern.

9   B D

During pregnancy, fasting plasma glucose concentration is decreased, probably due to the haemodilution effect of the increased plasma volume. The glomerular filtration rate is increased in normal pregnancy; this may lead to the renal threshold being exceeded and to glycosuria without impaired glucose tolerance. Fasting plasma insulin concentration rises in late pregnancy to accompany the increased glucose requirements. Glucose tolerance alters during pregnancy; although plasma glucose levels should have returned to normal two hours after an oral glucose load, insulin concentration frequently remains elevated.

10   A B C D

The amnion is derived from the blastocyst and is surrounded by the chorion. It is separated from its fellow by the chorion in a dizygous twin pregnancy. If one chorion only is present the pregnancy is monozygous. If a double chorion is present, the pregnancy may be either mono, or dizygous. The amnion covers the fetal surface of the placenta. The chorion is in contact with the decidua and therefore separates during the third stage of labour.

11   B E

Prostaglandins are produced in the seminal vesicles of man, but also in other tissues such as kidney, lung and brain. They are modified hydroxyacids derived from prostanoic acid, and contain a cyclopentane ring. They are chemically related to the thromboxanes. Prostaglandins of the E series increase renin secretion. There is no conclusive evidence that they are responsible for luteolysis in man; the evidence is speculative therefore the answer must be false.

12   A B D

Human milk contains around 2% protein compared to 3.5% in cows' milk; the fat content is similar at around 4%. Little iron is present (0.1 mg per 100 g milk) although the fat-soluble vitamins A, D, E and K and thiamine, riboflavin, nicotinic acid, and ascorbic acid are also present in adequate amounts. The sodium content of colostrum is considerably higher than that of mature milk (90 mg per dl vs 15 mg per dl).

13   C E

The only vitamins synthesised in the body are vitamin D(skin) and nicotinamide from tryptophan; the rest must be supplied in the diet. Vitamin K is fat-soluble as are vitamins A, D and E. Pyridoxine deficiency is very rare, occurring chiefly in children, producing convulsions and dermatitis. Naturally occurring folates are polypeptides containing 3, 5, 7 or more glutamic acid residues (polyglutamates). Vitamin D is cumulative, and excessive intake may cause renal failure (25-hydroxycholecalciferol is converted in the kidney to 1,25-dihydroxycholecalciferol).

14   C D E
The pudendal nerve arises from S2, S3 and S4.

15   A B D
Glucagon secretion is increased in diabetes mellitus, particularly in diabetic ketoacidosis (its main action is to raise the plasma insulin concentration). Insulin increases the rate of glucose utilisation in skeletal muscle, therefore in diabetes mellitus uptake is reduced. Insulin appears not to facilitate glucose uptake in brain, renal tubules, red blood cells and intestinal mucosa. The glucocorticoids enhance gluconeogenesis, secretion therefore is only increased in severe diabetic ketoacidosis.

16   A B D
Human placental lactogen is a polypeptide hormone immuno-logically and chemically similar to pituitary growth hormone. It is produced by the syncytiotrophoblast of the placenta and is detectable 12-18 days after fertilisation which closely follows the LH peak; increasing values are seen 35 days after the last menstrual period reaching a plateau at 34-36 weeks of pregnancy. Values obtained in the serum of mothers with multiple pregnancies are consistently higher. HPL is diabetogenic in that it is an antagonist of insulin; this results in an increase in circulating glucose. HPL also mobilises free fatty acids from fat depots.

17   B D
The main supporting structures of the uterus are the transverse cervical and utero-sacral ligaments. The round ligaments may assist in maintaining the uterus in anteversion but do not support it. The broad ligaments consist of twin folds of peritoneum without any supporting function.

18   A B D
Chylomicra are readily observed in lymph and plasma sampled three to four hours after a meal rich in fat. They are particles consisting mostly of triglycerides with some cholesterol, phospholipid and protein; they would not normally be present in the plasma of a person who has fasted twelve hours or more. In the fasting state free fatty acids are adsorbed to plasma albumin.

Cholesterol is predominantly contained in the low density lipoprotein fraction (ß fraction on electrophoresis). The high density fraction contains approximately 19% cholesterol compared to 47% for the low density. Free fatty acids are the form in which lipid is transported in the blood from adipose tissue deposits. The levels rise in the fasting state and during prolonged muscular exercise.

19 C
Mumps virus accounts for 10% of all cases of aseptic meningitis and meningoencephalitis, but is the only one of the named viruses to do so.

20 A C E
Occasionally almost the whole of the mesonephric duct persists and is then known as Gartner's duct. The epoophoron and paroophoron arise from Wolffian remnants. The processus vaginalis is a diverticulum from the coelomic cavity, it becomes a herniation of peritoneum into the scrotum to receive the descending testis. The round ligament is of mesodermal origin.

21 E
Oestriol production and excretion far surpasses that of oestrone and oestradiol; oestriol is the characteristic oestrogen of pregnancy, being produced by the 'feto-placental unit', hence its value as a monitor of placental function. There is marked increase in the renin-angiotensin system, hence an increase in aldosterone. HCG, produced by the trophoblast, reaches its peak during the first trimester of pregnancy (normally at approximately 10 weeks). The average urinary excretion of androgens in pregnancy has been shown to be no different from that in the non-pregnant woman. There is an increase in serum protein-bound iodine.

22 A
B. anthracis is a Gram-positive, aerobic, spore-bearing bacterium. *Cl. welchii* is Gram-positive but is an anaerobe; spores are never found in the tissues and only rarely seen in culture. *Ps.aeruginosa* is a Gram-negative non-spore-bearing rod. *C. diptheriae* is a Gram-positive but non-spore-bearing rod. *Cl. botulinum* is spore-bearing but a strict anaerobe.

23 A D
In the female, the sex chromosomes are normally XX. Barr observed that a large proportion of interphase nuclei from female tissues contained a characteristic small condensed mass of chromatin often lying against the nuclear membrane. It is believed that all female cells contain the sex chromatin (Barr body). The Y

chromosome determines testicular development. Up to the seventh week of development the appearance of the external genitalia is similar in both sexes.

24   A C E
Megestrol and chlormadinone are 17-alpha hydroxyprogesterone derivatives.

25   B D
Chlorambucil and cyclophosphamide are alkylating agents; they interact with DNA. Anthracycline is an antibiotic. 6-mercaptopurine is an antimetabolite, whose mode of action is to interfere with nucleic acid synthesis. Vinblastine (a vinca alkaloid) arrests cells in metaphase of mitosis.

26   A C
Insulin is secreted by the beta cells of the Islets of Langerhans; the alpha cells secrete glucagon. Insulin promotes the uptake of glucose and its deposition as glycogen in skeletal muscle. It also increases the rate of glucose utilisation in tissues. Glucose-6-phosphatase is only present in the liver, with a little in the kidney. Lactate is the end point of anaerobic metabolism of glucose. Adrenaline activates the enzyme adenyl cyclase and leads to the formation of 3'5'-cyclic AMP. This activates the enzyme phosphorylase kinase which in turn catalyses the conversion of inactive to active phosphorylase. This latter leads to breakdown of liver glycogen.

27   B C E
Lactic acid is the end product of anaerobic metabolism of glucose. There are a number of intermediate steps before glucose is oxidised by NAD+. NAD+ is produced from NADH+ by oxidation via the (respiratory) flavoprotein, cytochrome chain. The reaction occurs in the mitochondria. The energy produced in the reaction is stored as ATP (via pyruvate and acetyl CoA).

28   A C E
The mitosis sequence is interphase-prophase-metaphase-anaphase-telophase. Crossing-over occurs in anaphase of meiosis. Anaphase describes the phase at which the centromere of each chromosome divides and each member of a pair of chromatids moves along the spindle to opposite poles of the cell. Lag may occur in the process but the mechanism is not known. Both metaphase and telophase take longer than prophase in mitosis, although prophase is prolonged in meiosis. Replication of DNA is the purpose of mitosis.

29   B C E

There is no absorption nor reabsorption in the oesophagus or ureter. There is both absorption and secretion in the duodenum, although the jejunum and ileum are the main sites of absorption. Water absorption is completed in the colon, having started in the small intestine. The collecting tubules of the kidney are the sites of water diffusion from collecting ducts into hypertonic medullary interstitium, enabling the urine to become progressively more concentrated (in response to antidiuretic hormone).

30   A C D E

The cervix undergoes cyclical changes during the menstrual cycle; in particular, the amount of mucus, secreted by the cervical glands alters. Columnar epithelium lines the canal and meets squamous epithelium at the squamo-columnar junction. This junction may lie in the canal or on the ectocervix (ectropion), therefore in the latter circumstance glands may open onto the vaginal surface. Only the lining of the endometrial cavity is shed at menstruation. Peritoneum is reflected onto the posterior aspect of the supravaginal cervix.

31   A B C

A linear increase in serum cholesterol level takes place from early pregnancy until the last month, when the level forms a plateau. Serum alkaline phosphatase activity rises markedly in pregnancy (and has been used as a test of placental function). Levels of aspartate aminotransferase and alanine aminotransferase do not increase above the non-pregnant level in normal pregnancy. Clotting time and bleeding time are unchanged.

32   E

The menopause is occurring later than formerly. It is associated with decreased bone density due to demineralisation. Vaginal acidity is decreased due to loss of glycogen from the epithelial cells. Oestrone becomes relatively increased over oestradiol, the production of which falls markedly. The uterine body atrophies to a greater extent than the cervix.

33   B E

The upper part of the rectum is covered with peritoneum in front and at the sides; the middle part is covered in front only; the lower part lies below the level of the recto-vaginal pouch and therefore is devoid of peritoneal covering. Blood supply is from the inferior mesenteric artery through its rectal branches. Transverse folds project into the lumen consisting of mucous membrane and circular smooth muscle. Appendices epiploicae are not found in association with the rectum and taeniae coli are associated with the colon only.

34   A B C
Cystic fibrosis is transmitted as a recessive gene, as is phenylketonuria. It is believed that in certain parts of the world as many as 1 in 10 of the population carries the mutant gene for thalassaemia. There is an increased familial incidence of congenital pyloric stenosis probably due to a genetic origin, but the mode of inheritance is not known. Likewise Hirschsprungs' disease is thought to be at least partly genetically determined, but the mode is unknown.

35   A E
The diameter of the jejunum is greater than that of the ileum. The valves become less frequent in the jejunum and disappear in the terminal ileum. There is gradual decrease in villus size from pylorus to the ileo-caecal valve. Brunner's glands are almost exclusively found in the duodenum.

36   B C
The cytotrophoblast lies deep to the syncytiotrophoblast, retains the capacity to multiply and represents an inactive layer which can be stimulated to replace damaged or destroyed syncytio-trophoblast. An electron-dense mucoprotein layer ('fibrinoid') separates fetal and maternal tissue. It is suggested that this layer is involved in immunological 'protection' for trophoblast cells. Iron is stored in trophoblast tissue. Placental septa are probably of maternal origin. The number of stem villi decreases with advancing gestation.

37   A E
Juxtamedullary nephrons have much longer loops than outer cortical nephrons. The afferent arteriole is the thicker (and thus sensitive to angiotensin II). The junction between the ascending limb of the loop of Henle and the distal convoluted tubule is the site of the macula densa.

38   C D
The round ligament is 10-12 cm long. It is a fibromuscular cord (smooth muscle) passing from the lateral angle of the uterus in the anterior layer of the broad ligament to the internal inguinal ring. Along with the ovarian ligament it is the pathway along which the female gonad might have descended to the labium majus; it runs anteriorly to the obturator artery and passes lateral to the inferior epigastric artery.

39 D E

The adrenal cortex and medulla have separate embryological origin, the cortex being derived from mesoderm and the medulla from ectoderm. The average weight of the normal adult gland is 4 grams (range 2-6 g). Each gland is supplied by three separate arteries but drained by a single vein. The zona reticularis lies next to the medulla and produces cortisol; aldosterone is predominantly synthesised by the cells of the zona glomerulosa.

40 B D

Eccrine glands are commonest; apocrine glands occur in axilla, pubic region and areolae of breasts. The arrectores pili muscles pass obliquely from the epidermis to the slanting surface of the hair follicles deep to the sebaceous glands. By contracting, they cause the hairs to stand erect, and lead to the release of sebum. Split-skin grafts consist of epidermis, dermis and the superficial layers of the corium; regeneration takes place from hair follicles and sweat ducts. Melanocytes lie in the deepest layer of the epidermis. Melanin results from the enzymatic oxidation of tyrosine by tyrosinase, which is attached to the melanocytes at the epidermo-dermal junction. Corpuscles of Ruffini are thought to be heat receptors.

41 B

The median of a series of observations is the centre value when the observations are ranged in order from highest to the lowest. The sum total of values divided by the number of observations is the mean. The value occurring most often is the mode or modal value. The distance between the highest and lowest values is the range. The square root of the standard deviation has no specific meaning.

42 A B D

The lesser sac is the extensive pouch lying behind the lesser omentum and the stomach and projecting downwards between the layers of the greater omentum; the sac is anterior to the transverse mesocolon. The hepatic artery is one of the three branches of the coeliac trunk and swings to the right along the upper border of the pancreas to the front of the portal vein. Therefore the sac lies anterior to the artery and the pancreas. The foramen of Winslow is where the right extremity of the sac opens into the main peritoneal cavity. The boundaries are as follows:

Anteriorly	The free edge of lesser omentum containing the common bile duct to the right, hepatic artery to the left and portal vein posteriorly.
Posteriorly	The inferior vena cava.

Inferiorly	The first part of the duodenum.
Superiorly	The caudate process of the liver.

43   A D E

The primary branches of the coeliac axis are the hepatic artery, the splenic artery, and the left gastric artery. The gastro-duodenal artery is a branch of the hepatic artery and therefore not a primary branch of the coeliac axis. The right gastro-epiploic artery is a branch of the gastro-duodenal artery.

44   A C E

The sequence is vein, artery, nerve, going from medial to lateral. The femoral ring is the internal orifice of the femoral canal. It is bounded anteriorly by the inguinal ligament and posteriorly by the pectineal line of the pubis. The ring itself is normally occluded by a pad of tissue containing a lymph gland only. The inferior epigastric artery runs medial to the deep inguinal ring, hence the value of the artery in differentiating indirect (lateral to artery) from direct (medial to artery) inguinal herniae.

45   B E

A synovial joint consists of two ends of bone capped with hyaline cartilage and enclosed by an articular capsule. This consists of a fibrous capsule and a synovial membrane which produces the synovial fluid to keep the surfaces lubricated. The patello-femoral joint is a good example. The sacro-iliac joints are the articulations between the auricular surface of the sacrum and ilium on each side; they are synovium-lined and cartilage-covered joints. The sacro-coccygeal and lumbo-sacral joints are intervertebral (symphysis) joints; their surfaces must be firmly bound to provide strength for their supporting function. Adjacent bodies are covered by a fibro-cartilagenous disc (annulus fibrosus); the centre of the disc is filled with fibrogelatinous pulp (nucleus pulposus), with no joint cavity. Each pubic bone is covered by a layer of hyaline cartilage, and connected across the midline by a dense layer of fibro-cartilage.

46   A B

The deep perineal nerve innervates the urogenital diaphragm and the three superficial perineal muscles; it also sends twigs to levator ani and external sphincter ani. The pudendal nerve runs through the lesser sciatic notch anterior to the sacro-tuberous ligament and posterior to the sacrospinous ligament. The skin of the anal triangle is supplied by the inferior rectal nerve (S3,4) the perineal branch of S4 and some twigs from the coccygeal plexus (S5). The obturator nerve arises from the lumbar plexus (L2,3,4).

47 A B C E

Red marrow is present in the bones of the vault of the adult skull. The red cell nucleus is extruded at the normoblastic stage. Lymphocytes are normally formed in the lymphoid tissue of the bone marrow, thymus, spleen and lymph nodes. Normal megakaryocytes are polyploid. Megakaryocyte abnormalities may include small mononuclear or binuclear forms.

48 A

Clostridia are strict anaerobes. *Cl. tetani* produces terminal spores ('drumstick' appearance). Gas gangrene organisms include *Cl. septicum, histolyticum, sporogenes* and *bifermentans. Cl. welchii* is often a vaginal commensal organism, therefore it is not necessary to treat actively when isolated on vaginal swabs. Barrier nursing is not necessary because Clostridia are endogenous microbes and the infections which they cause are not contagious.

49 C

T. pallidum cannot be Gram-stained but can be demonstrated by a silver impregnation method. The primary chancre appears 9-90 days following infection. In tertiary syphilis 10-20% of cases give negative reactions. The WR test is not specific for syphilis; yaws, pinta and bejel give positive reactions, and false-positive reactions may occur in malaria, leprosy, glandular fever, smallpox vaccination and pregnancy. The treponemal immobilisation test is more reliable, but technically difficult. A living suspension of *T. pallidum* is incubated under anaerobic conditions in the presence of complement and patient's serum, and observed under dark-ground illumination, where the spirochaetes are rendered non-mobile, in positive cases.

50 A B D E

Cytomegalovirus is a herpesvirus, a group that also includes herpes simplex virus and varicella. At least 80% of adults have been infected, and the proportion may be as high as 95%. Most are asymptomatic, but latent infection may occur, especially in salivary glands. Infection in utero may lead to cytomegalic inclusion disease, a fatal generalised illness characterised by jaundice, haemolysis, and hepatosplenomegaly.

51 A B E

H. influenzae is an important cause of meningitis especially in young children. Acute meningococcal meningitis is fairly common; it often occurs in epidemics. It is preceded by infection of the nasopharynx and simple bacteraemia. Pneumococci are present in the throat of a large proportion of normal people and may occasionally lead to acute meningitis. *Staphylococcus albus* is not normally pathogenic and β haemolytic *Streptococcus meningitis* is very rare.

52 C

The pronephros represents a primitive form of kidney in certain mammals. In man this form of excretory apparatus is rudimentary, but acts as an organiser for the mesonephric ducts. Normal development of paramesonephric ducts may occur in the presence of streak gonads. The ova originate in the yolk sac wall and migrate via the innermost layer of the dorsal body wall and thence into the developing genital ridge. At least part (possibly all) of the vagina is formed from the urogenital sinus. Sexual differentiation is not complete before the tenth week of life.

53 A E

Both maxilla and mandible are derived from the first pharyngeal arch; the tonsil is derived from the second pouch, the thymus from the third. The anterior lobe of the pituitary does not derive from a true pharyngeal pouch, but from the ectoderm of the stomodeum (Rathke's pouch).

54 B

Haemophilia is inherited as a sex-linked recessive condition. Therefore sons of an affected male are unaffected, as they inherit the Y chromosome. Half of the sons of a carrier female will inherit the condition (one of the X chromosomes in the carrier female carries the gene). Similarly half the daughters of a female carrier will inherit a normal X chromosome from both parents. Because the gene is recessive, all daughters born to an affected male and normal female will be carriers. To exhibit the disease both X chromosomes would require to carry the gene (as would occur if parents were a haemophiliac male and a carrier female). However, an affected male and carrier female have a 50% chance of producing a normal male offspring.

55 B C D

The majority of immunoglobulins are gamma-globulins but there is some electrophoretic activity in the alpha and beta regions. The classes resemble each other in that the molecules are composed of two identical light polypeptide chains and two identical heavy chains. The difference lies in their heavy chains. However, in any one class there are two types, differing in the light chains. IgG is of sufficiently low molecular weight to cross the placenta. The first-formed antibodies are of the IgM type; IgG appears later. IgE is present in extremely small amounts in plasma; it is the tissue antibody responsible for atopic hypersensitivity.

56 A
The mean is the sum total of values divided by the number of observations. The median is the centre value with the observations ranged in order from highest to lowest. With a normal distribution, the mean, median and mode coincide. 99.7% of the population lies within 3 standard deviations. The standard error of the mean is the standard deviation divided by the square root of the number of observations. There are several other possible symmetrical distributions, including biphasic distribution and the uniform distribution.

57 A B C D E
Basal fetal heart rate varies with gestational age, partly because it is not subject to parasympathetic activity before the 20th week of pregnancy. The heart rate may accelerate with external head compression although bradycardia is more usual. An uncomplicated tachycardia is often a sign of maternal pyrexia. Atropine sulphate, by causing parasympathetic blockade leads to acceleration of the maternal and fetal heart rate.

58 C E
From midpregnancy onwards the fetal kidney increasingly contributes to amniotic fluid volume, contributing some 500 ml per day by term; in renal agenesis the liquor volume is greatly reduced. The volume of amniotic fluid may be estimated by ultrasound, but not accurately. Liquor volumes are higher than average in rhesus affected pregnancies, and grossly increased in hydrops fetalis. Amniocentesis may permit amniotic fluid to leak away, thus reducing the volume; it is not likely to increase it. Pre-eclampsia and intrauterine growth retardation are both associated with reduced amniotic fluid volumes.

59 A C D
In western societies arterial pressure tends on average to rise with age, but this trend is not apparent in the developing countries. The mechanism is likely to be decreasing compliance in the arterial system. Obesity and sedentary occupation are both factors which pre-dispose to elevated blood pressure. There is no evidence for a single gene mode of inheritance. There is no correlation with parity.

60 D E
Epithelioid cells are macrophages which phagocytose the tubercle bacilli. They are characterised by pale eosinophilic cytoplasm and elongated nuclei. Some macrophages may fuse to become so-called Langhans giant cells. Epithelioid cells become surrounded by a wide zone of lymphocytes and fibroblasts. Within 10-14 days

necrosis begins in the centre of the mass, this being a coagulative necrosis or caseation. Siderocytes are red cells containing haemosiderin, and they are increased after excessive iron intake.

ANSWERS TO PRACTICE EXAM 2

1   **A B E**
The cervical mucus at ovulation appears as a copious transparent fluid in contrast to the rest of the cycle when it is scanty and opalescent; the cervical mucus is alkaline. Fructose is a reducing sugar which provides the chief form of energy for spermatozoa under anaerobic conditions. There is no evidence that semen is 'sucked' into the uterus at intercourse. It is believed by some that a retroverted uterus with the cervix pointing towards the anterior vaginal wall may be a factor in infertility by reducing contact with the seminal pool.

2   **A B E**
IgG cytotoxic anti-sperm antibodies have been isolated from cervical mucus. Proteinase inhibitors are necessary to avoid digestion of the protein content of the spermatozoa. The mucus of midcycle is copious, clear and of egg-white consistency; it draws out into long strands without snapping ('Spinbarkeit'). However, these appearances merely confirm adequate oestrogen stimulation; they do not confirm ovulation. There are no changes characteristic of multiple pregnancy.

3   **B C D E**
Spermatogenesis, the formation of a mature sperm from a primitive germ cell takes approximately 70± 4 days in the human male. FSH acts directly upon Sertoli cells to facilitate spermatogenesis; a second requirement is for testosterone which is produced by the Leydig cells of the testis in the intertubular tissue under the influence of LH and then transferred into the tubular lumen. The 47XXY chromosomal pattern produces the syndrome of Klinefelter or seminiferous tubule dysgenesis. The external genitalia are normal male, as testosterone production is often sufficient for male secondary sexual characteristics to develop although the testes are usually small.

4   **B C E**
C-reactive protein is so-named because it reacts as a precipitate with the C-polysaccharide of pneumococcus. It is found in other infections also, and in rheumatoid arthritis, and following trauma.

Its appearance is closely related to a rise in ESR; both are therefore non-specific. The ESR is higher in normal women than in men, and it shows a significant rise with age. It is normally raised in malignant disease but its lack of specificity means it is of little value in monitoring the course of the disease. Any increase in the plasma content of high molecular weight substances is found to increase the ESR.

5   B D E
Prostaglandins are fatty acids, found in prostatic fluid but predominantly produced by the seminal vesicles. They induce rhythmic uterine contractions and are used for induction of labour or ripening the cervix. Prostaglandins tend to produce diarrhoea, not constipation. Aspirin acts by inhibiting the synthesis of prostaglandins, as the latter are thought to be responsible for inflammation, pain and pyrexia. Bronchospasm is rare, but may occur with PgF2$\propto$; care is therefore required in asthmatic patients.

6   C
There is no evidence that maternal growth hormone positively influences birth weight. Primiparity and social class are not consistently related to birth weight.

7   A C D
Intrauterine growth is determined by the genetic potential and the environment. The height and weight of the mother both exert a major influence on fetal weight; paternal factors influence the eventual size of the child but have little or no influence on intrauterine growth. Altitude may influence birth weight directly through its effect on the oxygenation of maternal and fetal circulation. An increase of 1000 m in altitude results in a decrease of about 100 g in birth weight. Intrauterine infections including cytomegalovirus are frequently accompanied by intrauterine growth retardation or even death. The maternal weight gain in pregnancy is not closely correlated with fetal growth being mainly due to maternal rather than fetal tissue. Maternal diabetes mellitus generally results in macrosomia rather than reduced fetal growth.

8   A D
Renin is a protein of molecular weight 65,000. It is mainly produced in the kidney but in small amounts in other tissues such as the uterus and salivary glands. Cells in the juxtaglomerular apparatus of the kidney are sensitive to changes in pressure in the afferent arteriole. A fall in blood pressure stimulates renin release which leads to production of angiotensin II and aldosterone. Aldosterone enhances reabsorption of sodium, and a decrease in blood sodium

concentration and/or a rise in potassium will stimulate aldosterone release. Potassium secretion in association with sodium reabsorption occurs in the distal tubular epithelium.

9   A B D
There are normally 4,000-11,000 white blood cells per ml of human blood. Monocytes are usually larger than other peripheral blood leucocytes. Only 1% of the polymorphonuclear leucocytes in females have a drum-stick appendage attached to one of the lobes; this may represent the inactive X chromosome. Lymphocytes do have a basophilic cytoplasm when mature. Eosinophils constitute only a very small proportion (<5%) of the white cell count under normal conditions. The packed cell volume is slightly lower in women being in the range 36-48%, compared to 40-52% seen in men.

10   A B
HCG is detectable in maternal serum around the time of implantation of the ovum at 5-6 days post-ovulation but within the present limitations of sensitivity of radioimmunoassay it has not yet been possible to demonstrate HCG prior to this time. Because of the close structural similarity between HCG and LH the two hormones are very similar in their biologic and immunologic properties. One of the major roles for HCG is its stimulus to sustain the functioning corpus luteum, converting it into the corpus luteum of pregnancy. There exists no evidence to implicate HCG in the initiation of parturition, maternal serum concentration altering little in late pregnancy. No association has been shown with pre-eclampsia.

11   A B C
HPL is a polypeptide hormone secreted by the syncytiotrophoblast of the placenta. It is immunologically and chemically similar to pituitary growth hormone with additional lactogenic properties. Maternal serum HPL concentration and placental weight do correlate but the link is not sufficiently close to permit fetal weight prediction. Serum levels of HPL do not vary much in relation to the time of day.

12   A C D
Biochemical tests demonstrate a rise in serum alkaline phosphatase concentration particularly towards the end of pregnancy. Serum total cholesterol is also raised but esterification is normal. There is a fall in the serum albumin concentration which is responsible for the fall in total proteins; however the serum globulin concentrations rise in pregnancy. Serum transaminase levels are unaltered.

13 A C E

The fetal zone of the adrenal cortex comprises approximately 80% of the gland in fetal life; after birth these cells undergo involution and disappear by 6 months of age. Human growth hormone is produced in utero by the fetal pituitary gland, maximal secretion occurring between 20 and 24 weeks. The fetus near term can respond to a glucose load by increasing the serum concentration of insulin but the response is usually small except in the offspring of diabetic mothers. The intermediate lobe of the pituitary gland is more prominent in the fetus than in the adult in whom it is not well represented or understood. Chromaffin cells, which contain noradrenaline, are found in the adrenal medulla, but also around the aorta, in the skin and throughout the alimentary tract. During fetal life and early childhood chromaffin cells are abundant. By the second year of life they atrophy but may be detectable for several years as the organ of Zuckercandl.

14 B D E

Oxytocin is a polypeptide consisting of eight amino acids. It is synthesised in the paraventricular nuclei of the hypothalamus. It passes down the axons of the pituitary stalk to reach the posterior lobe of the pituitary whence its release is controlled principally by nerve impulses from the hypothalamus. It differs in only two amino acid residues from vasopressin (antidiuretic hormone), also synthesised in the hypothalamus and stored in the posterior pituitary. Because of this, oxytocin has some antidiuretic properties. The uterus in early pregnancy is not very sensitive to oxytocin, but the latter may be used as a synergistic agent (with prostaglandin) in therapeutic abortion.

15 A C D

Progesterone is a steroid hormone which is formed in the ovary, placenta, adrenal gland and testis. All the steroid hormones are synthesised from acetate or acetyl co-enzyme A. The early synthetic steps are common to all steroids and involve the formation of cholesterol. Progesterone after secretion becomes largely bound to carrier plasma proteins. It is degraded mainly in the liver and a small fraction appears in the urine as the inactive conjugate pregnanediol glucuronide. The main source of 17-hydroxyprogesterone hormone in the menstrual cycle and in early pregnancy is the corpus luteum but after 6-8 weeks of pregnancy the vast majority of progesterone is elaborated by the placenta. In pregnancy and probably during the menstrual cycle one of its actions is to reduce the excitability of the myometrium.

16   C E
TRH is a tripeptide (pyroglutamyl-histidyl-proline-amide). Human molar thyrotrophin has a far higher molecular weight than pituitary TSH. The amount of T_4 in free form plasma is 4 times greater than T_3 but because the metabolic activity of the latter is 4 times that of T_4 the contributions of free T_4 and free T_3 would be approximately equal in biological activity. 0.024% of thyroxine is normally in the free form. Thyroxine-binding globulin is increased by exogenous oestrogens and pregnancy.

17   A B C D
Progesterone is able to promote the excretion of sodium, probably by antagonising the action of aldosterone on the distal renal tubule. Progesterone acts on secondary sexual organs only when they have been prepared by the action of oestrogens. Progesterone is formed in the ovary, placenta, adrenal gland and testis in man. It is a relaxant of smooth muscle in blood vessels, uterus and alimentary tract and possibly ureter. Arrhenoblastomas are usually androgen secreting tumours; tumours more likely to produce progesterone are luteal cell tumours and teratomas/chorionepitheliomas and occasionally granulosa cell tumours.

18   A B E
Aldosterone is principally synthesised by the cells of the zona glomerulosa. Cortisol is produced in the zona reticularis and is under control of ACTH, secreted by the basophil cells of the pars anterior of the pituitary gland. Aldosterone is not under direct ACTH control, but release is mediated through sodium levels via the renin-angiotensin system. The circadian rhythm is maintained by pituitary ACTH secretion and mediated by variation in corticotrophin-releasing factor secretion from the median eminence of the hypothalamus. The zona fasiculata forms the greater part of the cortex, and is probably a non-secretory zone of 'reserve' cells.

19   C D
Antimetabolites are 6-mercaptopurine (a purine antagonist) and methotrexate (a folic acid antagonist). Cyclophosphamide and thiotepa are alkylating agents. Actinomycin is an antibiotic.

20   A C D
Morphine depresses respiration by reducing sensitivity of the respiratory centre to rises in blood carbon dioxide tension; with high doses carbon dioxide narcosis may develop. The pupils constrict (due to third nerve muscle stimulation). Morphine impairs sympathetic vascular reflexes and stimulates the vagal centre. Orthostatic hypotension may therefore be a problem, particularly

in those taking antihypertensive drugs. Intrabiliary pressure may rise substantially, due to spasm of the sphincter of Oddi; biliary colic may therefore be aggravated by morphine. Morphine is conjugated in the liver (glucuronide) and excreted by the kidney.

21 A C D
The prostaglandins are a group of chemically related 20 carbon-hydroxy fatty acid derivatives of prostanoic acid. It seems likely that they are synthesised in most and possibly all organs of the body from arachidonic acid. The enzyme that converts arachidonic acid to acyclic endoperoxide is inhibited by indomethacin. PgE_2 augments platelet aggregation during coagulation. PgE_2 will also stimulate the smooth muscle of the uterus and is used as an abortifacient and inductor of labour. It is not an antidiuretic.

22 C D
Tetracycline has been shown to be selectively taken up by growing bones and teeth of the fetus, due to chelation with calcium phosphate. Chloramphenicol may cause neonatal death by circulatory collapse ('grey baby' syndrome). There is no evidence that sulphadimidine is harmful to the fetus. Sodium amytal is often used as a hypnotic in pregnancy. Ampicillin is currently the drug of first choice for the treatment of urinary tract infection in pregnancy. Whilst relatively few drugs have been shown to have teratogenic effects, there are many others whose effects on the fetus are uncertain. A good principle is to keep to an absolute mimimum the prescribing of drugs during pregnancy.

23 B C D E
Large amounts of histamine are found in the anterior and posterior pituitary lobes and the hypothalamic median eminence. The mast cells contain most of the histamine in the posterior pituitary gland although this is not the case in other sites. Histamine causes contraction of visceral smooth muscle but relaxes vascular smooth muscle and increases capillary permeability. Histamine is, in part, responsible for the wheal part of the triple response. Histamine also has a potent stimulatory effect on gastric acid secretion and is present in high concentration in gastric mucosa.

24 A B E
The commonest primary site for secondary ovarian tumours is the gastro-intestinal tract (particularly stomach and colon). These tumours are known as Krukenberg tumours; they are normally bilateral and may be true examples of transcoelomic spread. Breast cancer may occasionally metastasise to the ovary and is a fairly common cause of ovarian secondary tumours. Cervical cancer

tends to spread locally and does not metastasise to the ovary; hence it is not necessary to remove the ovaries when undertaking radical surgery for cervical cancer. Lung tumours spread commonly to the spine, brain and adrenal gland, but metastasis to the ovary is not common.

25   B C D

The Brenner tumour is an uncommon type of ovarian tumour and is grossly identical to a fibroma. Microscopically there is a markedly hyperplastic fibromatous matrix interspersed with nests of epithelioid cells. Brenner tumours are usually endocrinologically inert, but in recent years a number of cases have been associated with endometrial hyperplasia. Granulosa cell tumours commonly secrete oestrogen. Arrhenoblastoma is a functional description of an androgen secreting ovarian tumour; most commonly they show the histological pattern of Sertoli-Leydig cells, The very rare hilus cell tumour may secrete androgens.

26   A D

A cervical smear is a screening procedure; dyskaryotic squamous cells in a smear suggest the likelihood of dysplasia. Any smear containing such cells requires further investigation, by colposcopy and biopsy. Colposcopic findings dictate whether punch or cone biopsy is appropriate, to make an accurate diagnosis. Whatever form of treatment is felt appropriate, further cytology follow-up is mandatory.

27   A C

Breast carcinoma may be hormone-dependent. For this reason in metastatic breast cancer, hypophysectomy or oophorectomy is often undertaken with considerable palliation. There is no evidence that squamous cell carcinoma of the cervix is hormone-dependent although adenocarcinoma may be related to exogenous pro-gestogen intake (in the combined oral contraceptive pill). Normal cervical squamous epithelium is stimulated by oestrogen. Prostatic carcinoma was the first neoplasm of man to be successfully repressed by hormonal therapy. It is often androgen dependent; for this reason stilboestrol is very effective treatment. There is no evidence for hormone dependence in osteosarcoma or colonic carcinoma.

28   A B E

The dermoid cyst commonly contains ectodermal derivatives such as skin, hair follicles, and sebaceous or sweat glands. The tissues are mature and almost invariably benign. The nephroblastoma (or Wilm's tumour) is a malignant tumour of the kidney. Likewise the retinoblastoma is a developmental tumour of infancy and early childhood. The glioblastoma and reticulum cell sarcoma are derived from adult cells.

29   A C D E
Metastases are characteristic of malignancy. Malignant tumours tend to have a rapid rate of growth, but some grow more slowly than adjacent normal tissue (for example, some gut carcinomas). The presence of mitotic figures, particularly abnormal forms, is characteristic of malignancy. Malignant tumours tend to invade surrounding tissues (carcinoma of cervix is a good example). Loss of differentiation may be a feature of malignant tumours but a number of malignancies are characterised by well-differentiated tissue (for example, the mucus-secreting glands of well-differentiated adenocarcinoma of the cervix).

30   A B D
Tuberculoid reaction is characterised by epithelioid cells grouped together in follicles resembling those found in tuberculosis. Sarcoidosis is an example of a non-caseating tuberculoid reaction, also seen in leprosy. Crohn's and rheumatoid disease are other examples of a tuberculoid (or delayed hypersensitivity) type reaction. The chancre of primary syphilis exhibits a dense infiltration of lymphocytes, plasma cells and a few macrophages. Hashimoto's thyroiditis shows lymphocytic infiltration only.

31   A B D
The uterine artery anastamoses with the ovarian artery and the contralateral uterine artery. There is free communication between the branches of the external carotid arteries on each side (it is possible to ligate the common carotid artery for intra-cranial aneurysm arising on the internal carotid). The retinal, renal, and splenic arteries have no collateral circulations.

32   A B D
Phaeochromocytoma is a rare cause of hypertension. Tumours arising in the adrenal medulla usually secrete both noradrenaline and adrenaline while those originating in extra-adrenal chromaffin tissue secrete chiefly noradrenaline. Over 90% of tumours are benign. The greatest incidence is seen in the third and fourth decades. Although paroxysmal or sustained hypertension is the most common presentation a small number of patients display profound paroxysmal hypotension and tachycardia or alternating hypotension and hypertension.

33   D E

The Fallopian tube exhibits four types of epithelial cell, ciliated, secretory, intercalary (or peg) cells, and basal cells probably used in regeneration. Ciliated cells are most numerous in the region of the infundibulum and ampulla, with secretory cells more often found in the isthmus. There are three muscle layers. The fertilised egg remains in the tube for three or four days. The epithelium exhibits cyclical variation in response to oestrogen and progestogen levels; an optimum ratio is thought to be required to ensure passage onwards of the oocyte towards the uterus. There is no clear demarcation between the isthmus and ampulla.

34   A B D

There are rich venous communications with the dorsal veins of the clitoris. Lymphatic systems cross-connect (contralateral groin nodes may be affected by a tumour of the labium majus).

35   C E

The ureter is lined with transitional epithelium and has three muscle layers only. It passes down the psoas muscle crossing the bifurcation of the common iliac artery. From here it passes below the uterine artery to cross the lateral fornix of the vagina and enter the bladder in front of the vagina. The ureter possesses a longitudinal anastamosing network of arteries derived from the renal artery and aorta above, and the gonadal and vesical arteries below; it is of mesodermal origin.

36   A B

The trigone is relatively fixed and non-distensible. The ureters pierce the muscle and mucosal walls obliquely. The epithelium of the trigone arises from mesoderm.

37   A B E

The ischial spines are on the posterior border of the ischium, and demarcate an upper (greater) and lower (lesser) sciatic notch. They are normally not particularly prominent in the female pelvis; if they are they may lead to reduction of the interspinous diameter and arrest of the fetal skull. When the head is at the level of the spines, it is deeply engaged.

38   A E

The right ovary receives its blood supply from the abdominal aorta, the ovarian artery arising at the level of the renal arteries. The veins on the right side drain to the inferior vena cava, but on the left, to the left renal vein. The ovary is attached to the back of the broad ligament by the mesovarium. The lower pole of the ovary is attached to the lateral margin of the uterus by the ovarian ligament. There is no peritoneal covering of the ovary in the adult.

39   A D
The uterine artery passes above the ureter in the broad ligament (think of 'water under the bridge'). It supplies the cervix via a descending branch. It forms an anastomosis with the tubal branch of the ovarian artery. The round ligament is supplied by the ovarian artery in the broad ligament and by the inferior epigastric artery in the inguinal canal.

40   A B C D
The internal iliac artery is a terminal branch of the common iliac artery. It has four visceral and seven parietal branches:
Visceral   1.   Superior vesical a.
          2.   Uterine a. supplies vagina, uterus and tubes and anastomoses with the ovarian artery which arises directly from the aorta.
          3.   Middle rectal a.
          4.   Vaginal a. supplies vagina, bladder and ureter.
Parietal   1.   Umbilical a. obliterates soon after birth.
          2.   Obturator a.
          3.   Internal pudendal a.
          4.   Inferior gluteal a.
          5.   Superior gluteal a.
          6.   Lateral sacral a.
          7.   Iliolumbar a.

41   A D E
The pudendal nerve is part of the sacral plexus and arises from sacral nerve roots S2,3 and 4. It enters the gluteal region through the greater sciatic foramen on the medial side of the corresponding vessels. After crossing the ischial spine the nerve re-enters the pelvis through the lesser sciatic foramen. The pudendal nerve gives off the inferior rectal nerve and ends by dividing into the perineal nerve and the dorsal nerve of the clitoris (penis).

42   A B D
The femoral nerve arises from the posterior divisions of the 2nd, 3rd and 4th lumbar nerves. It descends in the groove between iliacus and psoas, passes deep to the inguinal ligament and enters the thigh on the lateral side of the femoral artery which in turn is lateral to the femoral vein. The femoral sheath is a tube-like continuation of the extraperitoneal fascia into the thigh; the aorta and its branches along with the inferior vena cava and its tributaries lie within the

fascial envelope while the spinal nerves emerge from the intervertebral foramina behind it.

43 A B D E

The inguinal canal is an oblique tract through the anterior abdominal wall. It extends from the deep inguinal ring, a deficiency in the transversalis fascia just above the midpoint of the inguinal ligament to the superficial inguinal ring, a deficiency in the external oblique aponeurosis, lying just above the pubic tubercle. The anterior wall is formed by the external oblique aponeurosis and additionally laterally by the internal oblique. The posterior wall is formed by transversalis fascia throughout with the conjoint tendon medially. The canal is traversed by the spermatic cord in the male and the round ligament in the female.

44 B D E

Physiological jaundice in a healthy baby appears after the first 48 hours of life, reaches a peak by about the fourth day and disappears within 7-10 days. The bowel is usually sterile at birth but is rapidly colonised by organisms including those encountered along the birth canal and perineum. Urine is seen to be passed in utero on ultrasound and is frequently passed at or soon after birth. The respiratory rate is usually less than 60 per minute at rest, 25-35 being usual. Constriction of the ductus arteriosus is brought about by the direct effect on the vessel wall of raising the arteriolar pO_2 with ventilation of the lungs at birth. There is probably a rapid partial closure soon after birth followed by a more gradual closure during the course of several days.

45 A B D

The superior surface of the sphenoid bone is indented to form the pituitary fossa (sella turcica); anterior is the shallow optic groove in which the optic nerves run. The optic chiasma is superior and posterior to the stalk; thus a tumour of the gland usually passes in front of the chiasma pressing on the medial sides of the optic nerves causing hemianopia of temporal fields. The two cavernous sinuses lie on either side. The pituitary gland receives its blood supply from the internal carotid artery and vessels in the tuber cinereum. The gland is all ectodermal in origin; Rathke's pouch (a midline ectodermal diverticulum from the stomodeum) forms the anterior lobe and the posterior lobe develops as a diverticulum from the floor of the diencephalon.

46 B C D

There are two distinct types of herpes simplex, 1 and 2. Herpes virus hominis type 2 causes herpes genitalis and vulvovaginitis and may lead to neonatal herpes because of transplacental transmission. The primary infection is usually subclinical, the virus remaining latent in the cells of the host. The virus may be transmitted during the 2nd stage of labour; for this reason the presence of active herpetic lesions is considered by many to be an absolute indication for delivery by Caesarean section. There appears to be no evidence that pregnancy per se leads to exacerbation of the condition, but other infections, sunlight, cold, and even menstruation may do so.

47   A C D
The Clostridia organisms consist of anaerobic Gram-positive bacilli which form spores that, in most cases, distend their bodies. They are widely distributed in nature as soil saprophytes and intestinal commensals of mammals. They include the causative organisms of botulism, tetanus, gas-gangrene and several intestinal infections. Their actions are typically mediated by endotoxins such as the powerful neurotoxin of *Clostridium tetani*.

48   D E
Treponema pallidum is purely a pathogenic parasite of man except under experimental conditions in apes, monkeys and rabbits. It is transmitted across the human placenta and thereby causes congenital syphilis. Being difficult to stain and of low refractibility it is best seen by dark ground microscopy. It cannot easily be grown on laboratory cultures. Yaws is caused by *T. pertenue* which is indistinguishable from *T. pallidum* in morphology, in serological reactions and in response to treatment.

49   A C
Streptococci are all Gram-positive but they may be aerobic or anaerobic. They are spherical or oval cocci with a tendency to form chains rather than clusters. If *S. viridans*, a normal commensal of mouth and pharynx, gains access to the blood stream, particularly during dental filling or extraction, in patients with existing heart disease they can cause subacute bacterial endocarditis. Staphylococci are the organisms which produce coagulase.

50   A C D
Alpha-fetoprotein is synthesised in the yolk-sac, the fetal liver and the fetal gastrointestinal tract early in pregnancy. Amniotic fluid levels follow the same trend as fetal serum levels. However, in maternal serum AFP concentrations show a very different pattern; there is a gradual rise up to 34-36 weeks of pregnancy after which there is a gradual decline to term and a very rapid drop after delivery. There is little correlation between maternal serum levels and amniotic fluid concentration. Elevation of the maternal serum

AFP is seen in twins, open neural tube defects, exomphalos and congenital nephrosis. Intrauterine death, where the normal integrity of the placenta (which blocks the transfer of AFP) is lost, also results in a rise in AFP. No rise has been demonstrated in association with congenital heart disease and microcephaly.

51　A E

Rhesus isoimmunisation is less common in ABO incompatible pregnancies as fetal red cells in the maternal circulation are coated with antibody much more quickly when ABO incompatibility exists and so sensitisation is less likely to be produced. 2-4% of Rh-ve women develop anti-D antibodies during their first pregnancy, but 25% of those mothers exposed to rhesus antigen will respond with antibody production. The commonest responsible rhesus antigen is D. The antigen is usually an intrinsic part of the red cell membrane. Cell bound antibodies are not able to cross the placenta to inflict haemolysis on the fetus; the responsible antibodies are the IgG group.

52　A

The paramesonephric ducts of each side appear as invaginations of the coelomic epithelium into the mesenchyme lateral to the cranial extremity of the mesonephric duct. The caudal part of the female mesonephric ducts degenerate and may persist as the Gartner's ducts. The caudal part of the female Mullerian duct does not degenerate but fuses with its partner from the other side to form the utero-vaginal canal. The caudal tip of this canal eventually comes into contact with the dorsal wall of the urogenital sinus where it produces an elevation, the Mullerian tubercle. The utero-vaginal canal and cells derived from its lower end give rise to the epithelial lining of the uterus and possibly part of the vagina. Proliferation of the tip of the uterovaginal canal results in a solid vaginal cord which increases progressively the distance between the uterovaginal lumen and the urogenital sinus. The vagina is thought to develop from canalisation of the sino-vaginal bulbs and the hymen is the portion which persists to a varying degree between the dilated canalised fused sinovaginal bulbs and the urogenital sinus proper. The Mullerian tubercle is therefore much higher. Sertoli cells are derived from sex cord cells initially joined to and possibly originating from germinal epithelium, not primordial sex cells. While the testis begins to emerge morphologically after the 7th week, ovarian development is not apparent until after the 13th week.

53　A C D E

A trait transmitted as an autosomal recessive is expressed only in homozygotes, persons who have received the gene from both parents. Theoretically the offspring of carrier parents have a 1 in 4 chance of being affected; two will be heterozygous and phenotypically normal and one will be homozygous for the normal allele and phenotypically normal; the fourth will be affected. Males and females are equally likely to be affected. Since rare recessive genes are passed down in families, the risk of having affected children is higher if a carrier marries within the family group. A parent or a grandparent of an affected child may well be similarly afflicted.

54 B
The standard deviation is the square root of the variance and is a measure of the scatter of observations around the mean. The population or sample group of observations should have a normal or Gaussian distribution. The standard deviation is not used in calculating chi-square. One standard deviation each side of the mean encompasses 66% of observations and two standard deviations 95%.

55 A C D
Cardiac muscle fibres have their own spontaneous rate of discharge and rhythmicity. The sino-atrial node, situated high in the wall of the right atrium near the entrance of the superior vena cava, has the highest rate and acts as the pacemaker. Sympathetic stimulation increases and the parasympathetic nerves decrease the heart rate. The parasympathetic nerve supply via the vagus nerve is predominant and lowers the heart rate to approximately 70/minute. Mesenteric traction causes a slowing of the heart rate by reflex vagal stimulation. Distention of the left ventricular wall causes a bradycardia through a parasympathetically-mediated effect.

56 C
The appearance of breast buds is the first evidence of sexual maturation in girls, who achieve puberty earlier than boys. Oestrogen treatment accelerates the rate of skeletal maturation. Mean maximum height velocity is 8-10 cm per year. The cervix is double the length of the uterus in the pre-pubertal period; the situation is reversed during adolescence.

57 D E
Haemoglobin A is a protein with a molecular weight of 64,450; the globin portion has alpha and beta chains. HbA2 contains alpha and delta chains. Haemoglobin F (fetal) is similar to HbA except that the beta chains are replaced by gamma chains. Fetal haemoglobin has the higher affinity for oxygen. Approximately 0.3g of

haemoglobin are destroyed and synthesised every hour (6g/day). Haem is an iron-containing porphyrin derivative.

58   D E

The absorption of ergometrine following intramuscular injection is unpredictable, and because of its local arteriospastic effect is certainly delayed in comparison to oxytocin; uterine contraction may not occur for up to five minutes following this route of administration. Because of this same arterioconstrictor effect acting generally following systemic absorption, hypertension may occur, and in pre-eclamptic patients this effect may lead to very marked elevation in blood pressure. Bradycardia and vomiting are common side-effects.

59   B C

Oxygenated blood returns from the placenta via the umbilical vein; the umbilical arteries carry deoxygenated blood from fetus to placenta. The ductus venosus provides a direct route of flow for oxygenated blood from the umbilical vein to the inferior vena cava. The foramen ovale connects the atria, and is an oblique passage through the interatrial septum, which closes soon after birth due to the greater left atrial pressure closing the septum premum against the septum secundum. The ductus arteriosus is a wide channel linking the left pulmonary artery with the aorta and joins the aorta distal to the origin of the three branches of the aortic arch.

60   C D

The presence of more than one cell line in an individual is mosaicism. Trisomy describes the presence of an extra chromosome. The buccal smear detects the presence of inactive X chromosome material; trisomy for the sex chromosomes (XXX or XXY) may therefore be detected, but trisomy involving the non-sex chromosomes or autosomes will not. Trisomy 21 is the commonest trisomy in live births, and it occurs with increasing frequency as maternal age rises (the risk being around 1 in 50 with maternal age in excess of 45 years). Rubella infection of the fetus in early pregnancy may lead to structural congenital malformations, but these are not due to chromosomal abnormality.

ANSWERS TO PRACTICE EXAM 3

1   A E
The oocyte and spermatozoa usually come together in the ampulla or outer third of the Fallopian tube. The full diploid genetic constitution is restored by fertilisation. At the early morula stage the conceptus is enclosed within the zona pellucida which is lost after the blastocyst stage. Oviductal cilia and possibly the musculature of the genital tract are the active transporters of the embryo rather than the morula itself. HCG can be detected by radioimmunoassay in maternal blood as early as 5 days after conception and in anticipation of implantation.

2   D E
The volume of amniotic fluid increases up to 36-37 weeks of pregnancy after which there is a decline. The pH of amniotic fluid is between 7.1 and 7.25 ie. alkaline. Organic constituents are mainly proteins and protein derivatives from maternal plasma. The protein content does decrease from 26 weeks onwards. A decrease in amniotic fluid volume is seen in pre-eclampsia and intrauterine growth retardation.

3   A B D E
Calcium homeostasis is maintained by three hormones: 1,25-dihydroxycholecalciferol which increases calcium absorption from the upper small intestine, parathyroid hormone which mobilises calcium from bones and increases urinary phosphate excretion, and calcitonin, a calcium lowering hormone which inhibits bone resorption. Calcium absorption is decreased by phosphates in the diet which bind to form insoluble salts with calcium. Fat soluble vitamins like D are poorly absorbed in the absence of pancreatic lipase; thus in pancreatitis deficiencies can develop. This may also result from coeliac disease. A high protein diet increases calcium absorption.

4   A B E
Subnuclear vacuolation of the glandular epithelium usually occurs 24-36 hours after ovulation. The changes which are seen in the endometrium after ovulation (secretory phase) are influenced by both oestrogens and progestagens. At the end of the secretory phase the walls of the spiral arteries constrict, causing ischaemia and necrosis of the endothelium. Rupture of the blood vessels above the constriction takes place and bleeding with desquamation of the functional layer of the endometrium occurs. Gland mitoses do continue to occur in menstruating endometrium. Subsequent to shedding, endometrial regeneration occurs from the zona basalis.

5   **A D**
Our understanding of the changes in cardiac output in pregnancy have evolved gradually with changes in measurement techniques. The most widely accepted view is that in the normal pregnant woman at rest, not lying supine, cardiac output rises from early pregnancy to a peak at around 20 weeks gestation which is approximately 1.5 litres per minute or 40% above the non-pregnant level; this level seems to be maintained throughout the rest of pregnancy. Although venous pressure in the legs has been shown to increase during pregnancy, that in the arms is unaltered, and central venous pressure is said to remain in the range 2-5 cm water. Peripheral resistance is calculated from the mean arterial pressure divided by cardiac output; since cardiac output is increased, and arterial blood pressure if anything falls slightly, it follows that peripheral resistance must be decreased. The fall has been estimated at between 20 and 40%, and seems to be maximal in mid-pregnancy; this is due to the opening up of new vascular beds within the uterus and placenta, and a general relaxation in peripheral vascular tone. The increased cardiac output of pregnancy is achieved by both an increase in heart rate (averaging 15 beats/min) and stroke volume (from 65 to 70 ml); again these changes are present from early pregnancy.

6   **A E**
Anatomically the ribs flare out in pregnancy long before there is any mechanical pressure; the subcostal angle changes from 68° to 80° by the 20th week. The diaphragm is raised and its excursion with respiration is greater. Airways resistance is reduced. The tidal volume, the volume inspired and exhaled at each breath, increases progressively throughout pregnancy and thus increases the minute ventilation as the respiratory rate remains unchanged. The vital capacity, the maximum volume of air that can be forcibly inspired after a maximum expiration, is probably unchanged although it has been suggested that there may be a slight increase (2% during the whole of pregnancy). Overall the total lung capacity is increased marginally.

7   **D**
Fibrinogen is synthesised in the liver and is responsible for blood coagulation. The concentration in plasma is markedly increased in pregnancy. The normal non-pregnant levels are in the region of 250-400 mg/100 ml in late pregnancy. The conversion of soluble plasma protein fibrinogen to insoluble fibrin is catalysed by thrombin. Vitamin K is necessary for prothrombin production; coumarin derivatives competitively inhibit vitamin K.

8 A D E

A normal diet would provide 12-15 mg iron daily. Ferric iron is not absorbed and must be reduced to the ferrous form before passing the gut wall; this reduction is assisted by ascorbic acid and sulphur-containing amino acids. Iron absorption is normally 10-15% but is increased if the body stores are reduced or the rate of formation of red cells is increased.

9 A B D E

The overall effect of aldosterone is to increase the amount of sodium in the body, its main action being to increase sodium absorption from the distal renal tubule and from the ascending limb of the loop of Henle and collecting ducts in exchange for potassium and hydrogen ions. Sodium retention is accompanied by water retention, increasing the extracellular fluid volume, and therefore total weight. Serum chloride level rises, in parallel with the sodium level.

10 D E

Fatty acids and monoglycerides are not water soluble; bile salts convert them to micelles, particles less than 0.5μm in diameter. Chylomicrons consist of cholesterol, phospholipid and protein and are the forms in which lipids accumulating in the cells pass out into the lymph. Dietary fat is absorbed in the upper part of the small intestine. The rate of cholesterol and myelin lipid synthesis is low in adult central nervous system. Fatty acids on oxidation yield a large quantity of energy. Linoleic acid is an essential fatty acid.

11 A B D

The net gain is two molecules of ATP (the remaining two are used for phosphorylation). Human growth hormone inhibits glucose uptake.

12 A C D

Active transfer of amino acids occurs to the fetus from the mother as fetal plasma levels are much higher for every amino acid. Water soluble vitamins are also actively transported in a similar way, but it is likely that fat soluble vitamins are transferred sluggishly by diffusion. Iron is actively transferred to fetus at the expense of the mother as is calcium also against the gradient but no gradient exists for magnesium, mother and fetus being in equilibrium.

13 B D E

Calcium is actively transported across the placenta to the fetus against a concentration gradient. Soon after birth the serum calcium concentration in the baby falls, maximally on the second day. Thereafter the level rises towards adult values during the next 2-3 days. It is therefore largely unrelated to maternal blood calcium at or around birth and is unlikely to be influenced by maternal dietary deficiency. Hypocalcaemia is seen in babies born to diabetic mothers and in association with neonatal hypoglycaemia. It does not usually cause permanent brain damage, but is a common cause of neonatal tetany and/or convulsions.

14 A B C
Prolactin is produced by the anterior pituitary, kept under tonic inhibition by secretion of a prolactin inhibiting hormone. Prolactin is secreted in the middle trimester of pregnancy, and increases progressively towards term. There is no fall just before delivery. On the contrary, levels rise further and are maintained as long as breast feeding continues. Prolactin has a very short half-life in the circulation. TRH may lead to both TSH and prolactin release.

15 C E
Thyroid-stimulating hormone is a glycoprotein. Thyroxine is tetraiodothyronine. The major action of thyroid hormones is to stimulate oxygen consumption. Cretinism may result from overtreatment of the mother with antithyroid drugs or severe maternal hypothyroidism. T_3 and T_4 are stored in the colloid vesicles of the follicles of the thyroid gland bound to thyroglobulin. Their release is stimulated by TSH. The inactive gland therefore shows an increased amount of colloid.

16 C D
Insulin is a polypeptide with two amino acid chains. It is produced by the β cells of the Islets of Langerhans; the α cells produce glucagon. Glucagon has a hyperglycaemic effect, and levels increase in response to hypoglycaemia. In the normal subject, insulin has a hypoglycaemic effect. Insulin is not required by exercising muscle to utilise glucose; it decreases glucose output from the liver and facilitates glycogen synthesis.

17 B C D E
Implantation is probably well underway by 5-6 days post-ovulation and HCG produced by the blastocyst to convert the corpus luteum in early pregnancy can be detected in maternal serum using a sensitive beta-HCG assay by 8 days post-ovulation. HCG rises rapidly in early pregnancy reaching a peak between 56 and 68 days after ovulation. Thereafter levels fall to 18 weeks after which they remain more or less constant until after delivery. HCG serves as the basis for most pregnancy tests. Pathologically high concentrations of HCG are seen in hydatidiform mole. Radioimmunoassy of HCG

in urine is used in the follow up of hydatidiform molar pregnancy and also to judge the efficacy of chemotherapy in chorioncarcinoma where it serves as an excellent tumour marker.

18   A C D E
The main function of parathyroid hormone is to regulate the concentrations of ionised calcium in body fluids, by its actions on bone, the small intestine and the kidneys. Excess parathyroid hormone enhances calcium mobilisation from bone producing hypercalcaemia. The destruction of the bone matrix is also enhanced causing an increase in plasma and urinary levels of hydroxyproline. Parathyroid hormone inhibits proximal tubular renal reabsorption of phosphate which leads to phosphaturia and hypophosphataemia. Parathyroid hormone also increases renal tubular reabsorption of calcium; however because the increase in the amount of calcium filtered overwhelms the effect on reabsorption there is a net increase in urinary calcium excretion.

19   C D E
The posterior pituitary gland secretes two hormones, oxytocin and arginine vasopressin. Both hormones are synthesised in the cell bodies of neurones in the supraoptic and paraventricular nuclei and transferred down their axons to the posterior pituitary. The principal physiological effect of oxytocin is on the myoepithelial cells of the breast ducts promoting milk ejection. Oxytocin also causes uterine smooth muscle contraction but it increases only once labour is established. Oxytocin is inactivated by oxytocinase produced by the placenta. Oxytocin has biological properties which overlap to some extent with vasopressin, in particular an antidiuretic effect.

20   B D E
Dehydration tends to increase rather than decrease the level of potassium in the plasma. Most of the potassium filtered by the kidney is reabsorbed in the proximal tubules and potassium is then secreted by the distal tubular cells. In the distal tubules sodium is generally reciprocally reabsorbed. In metabolic acidosis increased H^+ excretion by the kidney takes place, this reduces K^+ secretion and so plasma potassium is not decreased. Beta-cell tumours of the pancreas secrete insulin which promotes the intracellular passage of potassium reducing the plasma level. Thiazide diuretics act proximal to the distal tubule and increase sodium concentration in the distal tubular fluid and cause appreciable potassium loss in the urine. Individuals with primary hyperaldosteronism often become severely potassium depleted, probably by a similar mechanism.

21   E

The fetus has the enzyme systems necessary for the production of 3 β OH (delta 5) steroids such as pregnenolone and dehydro-epiandrosterone. The placenta is dependent on these precursors for the production of oestrogens; in order to do this it uses 3 enzyme systems which are not present in the fetal liver or adrenal, sulphatase, 3 β OH-steroid dehydrogenase, and aromatase. Thus maternal urinary oestriol excretion in pregnancy should be considered a measure of the synthetic properties of the feto-placental unit rather than of placental function alone. Oestriol excretion continues to rise steadily up to term, but thereafter plateaus. In fetal growth impairment, hypertensive disease, or other situations of fetal compromise, excretion may plateau or fall at an earlier stage. The decrease in excretion is a result of the deterioration in fetal condition, and there is no evidence that a fall in excretion may precede fetal compromise, e.g. by abruption. Excretion is not affected by maternal cardiac disease.

22   E

Fetal breathing movements detected by real-time ultrasound occur with a frequency of 50-60 breaths per minute. The proportion of time that is spent in breathing movements increases with gestation from around 10% at 28 weeks to 50% at term. Breathing activities also show a diurnal variation with 3 distinct patterns of periodicity: increasing 2-3 hours after maternal meals; increasing between 1 and 7 am; and increasing cyclically every 1-1.5 hours. Fetal breathing movements have also been found to occur for a reduced proportion of time in various disorders of pregnancy including growth retardation, antepartum haemorrhage, and pre-eclampsia.

23   A C D

The adrenal cortex secretes glucocorticoids, C21 steroids with widespread effects on the metabolism of carbohydrate and protein. The C21 steroids have both mineralocorticoid and glucocorticoid activity; mineralocorticoids are those with predominant effects on Na^+ and K^+ excretion and glucocorticoids are those which particularly affect glucose and protein metabolism. The two common glucocorticoids are cortisol and corticosterone, their actions including increased protein catabolism and hepatic glycogenesis and gluconeogenesis. Glucose-6-phosphate activity is increased and the blood glucose rises. Glucocorticoids inhibit ACTH secretion and ACTH secretion is increased in adrenalectomised animals. Adrenal insufficiency is characterised by an inability to excrete a water load and only glucocorticoids repair this deficit; the exact mechanism of glucocorticoid water excretion is contentious.

24 B C D E

The injectable anticoagulant heparin is a large molecule and does not cross the placenta as most oral anticoagulants do and is therefore the anticoagulant of choice in pregnancy. Tetracycline is contraindicated in pregnancy because it does cross the placenta. Adverse effects include deposition in and staining of deciduous teeth and bones, tooth malformations and decrease in linear bone growth. Sulphadimidine rapidly crosses from mother to fetus. If given immediately prior to delivery there is a theoretical risk of competition between sulphonamides and bilirubin for binding sites on neonatal albumin. Diazepam readily crosses the placenta whichever route of administration is used and can cause behavioural problems for many hours after birth if given in late pregnancy or labour. Salicylates cross the placenta and can cause neonatal platelet dysfunction, decreased neonatal factor XII, neonatal haemorrhage and respiratory distress syndrome.

25 A B C

Progesterone is a steroid hormone produced in the luteinised granulosa cells of the ovarian corpus luteum. During early pregnancy, between 5-7 weeks following the LMP placental trophoblast takes over progesterone production utilising cholesterol as the major precursor. It has a short half-life and is converted in the liver to pregnanediol, which is conjugated to glucuronic acid and excreted in the urine. Progesterone facilitates the secretory changes in the endometrium necessary for implantation of the fertilised ovum and it also acts as a smooth muscle relaxant hence suppressing uterine contractility.

26 A B E

Substances which mimic the action of progesterone may be called progestagens. Progesterone prepares the endometrium for implantation and maintenance of pregnancy. It therefore causes secretory changes in the endometrium, gland promotion rather than regression and it suppresses uterine excitability. It is progesterone which causes the loss of cervical mucus ferning after ovulation. Oestrogens rather than progestagens are thought to be responsible for the hypertensive implications of oral contraceptives. Progestogens reduce the permeability of cervical mucus to sperms.

27 A B D

The posterior pituitary gland produces two hormones oxytocin and arginine vasopressin. The principal action of vasopressin is reabsorption of water from the kidney and it is often called antidiuretic hormone. One of the physiological effects of oxytocin is on the smooth muscle-like cells of the breast ducts causing contraction and the squeezing of milk out of the alveoli of the lactating breast. Oxytocin also causes contraction of the smooth muscle of the uterus when its secretion is increased during labour. Ovulation is influenced by hormones of the anterior pituitary gland, follicle stimulating and luteinising hormones. Vasopressin and oxytocin do not appear able to affect placental growth, which is not thought to be directed by a specific hormone.

28   D E

Heparin is a high molecular weight polysaccharide present in the body primarily in mast cells in the lung and liver. It is the strongest organic acid in the body, and its strong electronegative charge in solution accounts for its anti-coagulant properties, acting largely as an anti-thromboplastin and an anti-thrombin. Heparin has a very short effective half-life in the circulation, and antagonists are rarely required in clinical practice. Nevertheless the strongly acidic nature of heparin means that protamine, a strongly basic protein, may be used for the more rapid reversal of heparin. Heparin limits the extension of established clot, but does not prevent embolisation. Thus the incidence of pulmonary embolism following heparinisation of patients with deep venous thrombosis is not greatly reduced, although the mortality rate associated with the condition certainly is.

29   A B C D E

These features are all characteristic of uterine fibroids, which are the commonest tumours in the female. The majority atrophy after the menopause, probably due to withdrawal of hormonal stimulation. Hyaline degeneration is the commonest type of degeneration in fibroids. Sarcomatous change is rare but occurs in approximately 0.1%. Calcification or 'womb stones' may occur and are detectable on plain X-ray. Red degeneration often occurs in pregnancy due to softening of the capsule and the increased blood supply.

30   A C D E

Blood supply to the endometrium comes from the radial and spiral arteries. Subnuclear vacuolation of the glandular epithelium is an early sign of ovulation occurring within 36 hours after ovulation. Endometrial glands already developed by oestrogen influence become tortuous under the influence of progesterone in the second half of the cycle and accumulate secretions. Glandular secretion reduces in the latter part of the secretory phase if conception does not occur. The walls of the coiled arteries constrict, closing off blood flow and producing ischaemia which leads to necrosis of the endometrium. The epithelial lining and the superficial portion of the lamina propria called the functional layer are sloughed during menstruation. The superficial compact and the deep spongy layers are noticeable before menstruation takes place.

31   A B D
The pituitary gland lies below and in front of the optic chiasma. The superior portion of the anterior part is known as the pars tuberalis. The anterior pituitary secretes six hormones: adrenocorticotrophic hormone, thyroid stimulating hormone, growth hormone, follicle stimulating hormone, luteinising hormone, all under the stimulation of the hypothalamus and prolactin controlled by an inhibiting factor. Few nerve fibres pass between the anterior pituitary lobe and the hypothalamus but there is a direct link via the portal hypophyseal vessels and releasing factors can thereby be transferred. Vasopressin and oxytocin are released from the posterior pituitary gland.

32   A C D E
Caudally the paramesonephric duct crosses the mesonephric duct to reach its medial side where it meets the duct of the other side in the urogenital septum. The two paramesonephric ducts eventually completely fuse in their lower part and the septum breaks down to form the uterovaginal canal. The caudal tip of the uterovaginal canal comes into contact with the dorsal wall of the urogenital sinus where it produces an elevation, the Mullerian tubercle. Throughout fetal and early postnatal life the cervical portion of the uterus is larger than the body and only alters in later life under hormonal influence. The caudal portion of the hind gut which receives the allantois is slightly dilated and called the cloaca; it is separated from the exterior by the cloacal membrane.

33   A C D E
The inguinal canal is an oblique tract through the anterior abdominal wall. It extends from the deep inguinal ring, a deficiency in the transversalis fascia just above the midpoint of the inguinal ligament to the superficial ingiunal ring, a deficiency in the external oblique aponeurosis, lying just above the pubic tubercle. The anterior wall is formed by the external oblique aponeurosis and additionally laterally by the internal oblique. The posterior wall is formed by transversalis fascia throughout with the conjoint tendon medially. The canal is transversed by the spermatic cord in the male and the round ligament in the female. The spermatic cord contains the ilioinguinal nerve. A prolongation of the peritoneum, the processus vaginalis, extends down the fetal inguinal canal and is later largely obliterated.

34 A B E
There are two main groups of lymph nodes in the lower limb, superficial and deep. The superficial group is divided into the upper sup. inguinal group which lies just below the inguinal ligament and drains lymph from the lower part of the abdominal wall, the perineum, external genitalia, anal canal and the gluteal region. The lower sup. group lies around the saphenous opening and drains lymph from the previous group of nodes and skin over the thigh, medial part of the leg and foot. The deep groups are found under the deep fascia in the popliteal and inguinal regions. The popliteal group drain the skin over the lateral side of the calf and foot. The deep inguinal group lie in the femoral canal and receive lymph from all the superficial nodes and deep vessels from the entire limb. Lymph drainage of the prostate is to internal iliac nodes. Lymph vessels from the testis pass to the para-aortic nodes in the region of the renal arteries.

35 B C E
The human pronephros is a transient phase of development represented by a few solid or vesicular cell groups derived from the intermediate mesoderm; its regression is complete by the beginning of the fifth week. Mesonephric elements differentiate from the nephrogenic cord. They divide at the cephalic end into a series of spherical masses, the mesonephric vesicles. The vesicles become pear-shaped; the lateral narrow part becomes tubular and unites with the mesonephric duct. The medial part of each mesonephric vesicle enlarges and its wall becomes invaginated by blood capillaries to form a glomerulus. The metanephros arises from the caudal part of the nephrogenic cord forming the metanephric blastema and from the ureteric outgrowth from the caudal part of the mesonephric duct, the ureteric bud. The nephrons develop from the blastema and the collecting system. The tubules, calyces, renal pelvis and ureter form from the ureteric bud. Urine formation begins about the third month of fetal life and continues in increasing volume to term. The mature fetus may well void 450 ml of urine daily into the amniotic cavity.

36 A B C D
A portal system is one which has a capillary plexus interposed on its pathway to the heart. The intestinal portal system serves a wide area including the entire alimentary tract from the lower end of the oesophagus to the upper part of the anal canal and the spleen, pancreas and gall bladder. The three major portacaval anastomoses are at the oesophagus, anal canal and umbilicus. The portal vein returns to the liver and divides repeatedly into a plexus of capillary sized vessels termed sinusoids; these empty into tributaries of the

113

large hepatic veins which emerge from the back of the liver and join the inferior vena cava. Drainage of the spleen is via the splenic vein into the portal vein and does not constitute a portal/systemic anastomosis.

37   B D
Congenital adrenal hyperplasia is an autosomal recessive disorder which is more often recognised in females, but is not truly X-linked as it is also seen in males. Classical achondroplasia is an autosomal dominant disorder. Hurler's syndrome is a severe autosomal recessive mucopolysaccharidosis (Hunter's syndrome is the X-linked disease). Duchenne muscular dystrophy and true hermaphroditism are both X-linked conditions.

38   A B E
Down's syndrome involves an excess of chromosome 21 material but in 4% of cases this does not amount to a separate chromosome. It most frequently arises due to non-separation of the chromosomes during meiosis. A female with Down's syndrome has a 1 in 2 chance of having a normal child. After the age of 40 the risk of an affected child is more than 1 in 100. Although the diagnosis of Down's syndrome should rest upon cytological culture from amniotic fluid and genetic studies, it is associated with reduced amniotic fluid alpha-fetoprotein.

39   A D E
Klinefelter's syndrome characteristically has an XXY chromosome complement. Cri du chat syndrome is apparently due to deletion of part of the short arm of chromosome 5. Patau's syndrome displays trisomy 13. Tay-Sach's disease is associated with a single autosomal recessive gene and achondroplasia is due to an autosomal dominant gene neither of which is normally recognisable without special techniques.

40   C
Chromosome studies of peripheral white blood cells usually require at least 72 hours of incubation. Colchicine is added to the medium to arrest mitosis at metaphase, by disrupting the mitotic spindle. It is in metaphase that chromosomes are most readily identified. Meiosis is a mechanism for reducing chromosome numbers, each daughter cell receiving half (23) the normal complement of 46 chromosomes.

41   E
In type IV cell-mediated immunity, sensitised lymphocytes come into contact with an appropriate antigen and release a number of

effector proteins, called lymphokines. These include migration inhibition factor, lymphotoxin, chemotactic factor, and interferon. They do not arise from mast cells or plasma cells, nor are they thought to be responsible for immune complex formation, but information on the subject of lymphokines is scanty at present.

42   A D E
Human leucocyte antigens are present on most nucleated cells. Two antigens are inherited from each parent making a total of four. Homozygosity may result in only two defined antigens being present but this is not the usual situation. In man, the transplantation antigens are determined by a number of genes situated at independent loci. The antigens determined by these gene complexes are termed the HLA antigens. It is thought that a combination of humoral and cellular factors is responsible for homograft rejection.

43   C D
IgG crosses the placenta providing the neonate with passive immunity. Immunoglobulins are also transferred to the baby in breast milk. Several transient neonatal diseases are the consequence of maternal IgG crossing the placenta, e.g. transient neonatal thyrotoxicosis. IgG and IgA appear in urine in pre-eclampsia and others in renal disease but not in normal pregnancy.

44   B C
Lymphocytotoxin is a protein substance liberated from T-lymphocytes stimulated by antigen. It is not found in all pregnant women; 10% of primigravid and 50% of multigravid women demonstrate lymphocytotoxic antibodies. There is no evidence to suggest that they cause fetal abnormalities or that they are associated with increased fetal wastage.

45   A D
The mean is the average, calculated from the sum of the value of the observations divided by the number of observations. The median is the central value of a series of observations, and is found by ranking the observations in order from the lowest to the highest value. The mode is the observation which occurs most frequently; in D therefore it is 2. They are all measures of central tendency and should coincide in normal symmetrical distribution. $P<0.05$ indicates that the probability of this result occurring by chance is 5 in 100 whereas with $P<0.01$ the likelihood is 1 in 100 and so the latter is the more significant. The scatter of observations around the mean is indicated by the standard deviation. The closer a sample size gets to the population as a whole the more likely are the two standard deviations to agree, but they are not the same. The prevalence of a

disease is the proportion of affected individuals in a population; the incidence is the frequency with which a disease occurs.

46   A C D E

The causative organism of bubonic plague, *Yersinia pestis*, is a flea borne pathogen of rats and other rodents. *Corynebacterium diphtheriae* is an obligate parasite and man is its only natural host; it is not naturally pathogenic to animals. *Bacillus anthracis* is mainly a pathogen of herbivorous animals such as cattle, sheep, goats, horses and camels. Human infection is usually cutaneous by direct contact with infected animal products or a severe haemorrhagic infection of the bronchi and lungs acquired by inhalation. Brucella organisms which cause undulant fever in man are primarily pathogenic to goats, cattle and pigs. Many of the leptospira are pathogens of animals such as rats, mice, dogs, cattle and pigs from which human infection originates.

47   B

Streptococcus viridans is a common inhabitant of the normal human throat. Transient bacteraemia may occur during eating or dental extraction. Usually these organisms are disposed of harmlessly but if there is a breach of the endothelial lining of the heart the organisms may cause subacute bacterial endocarditis. Staphylococci are usually responsible for paronychia. Beta haemolytic streptococci are commonly responsible for sore throats in children, acute nephritis and rheumatic fever.

48   A B D

Primary cytomegalovirus infection during pregnancy may affect both the placenta and the fetus in up to 50% of cases. The prognosis of the infection in the fetus is not accurately known, but it is thought that such infection may produce microcephaly, choroidoretinitis, eighth nerve damage, pneumonia, hepatosplenomegaly, anaemia (sometimes haemolytic with jaundice) and intrauterine growth retardation. Myocarditis and enterocolitis are not usually associated with CMV infection.

49   B C D E

Tay-Sach's disease is a form of gangliosidosis characterised by deficiency of hexosaminidase A activity, and transmitted as an autosomal recessive; the gene is carried by about 1 in 30 of the Ashkenazi Jewish population. Antenatal diagnosis is possible by assay of the enzyme in cultured amniotic fluid cells. Anencephaly, in common with other neural tube defects, is characterised by the finding of elevated levels of the oncofetal antigen alpha-fetoprotein in the amniotic fluid. Klinefelter's syndrome, the male form of sex chromosome trisomy, with the karyotype 47XXY, can be diagnosed by chromosomal analysis following culture of amniotic fluid fibroblasts.

Phenylketonuria is an inborn metabolic error due to a lack of the enzyme phenylalanine hydroxylase which usually converts phenylalanine to tyrosine. It is diagnosed post-natally by the presence of an alternative metabolic product, phenylpyruvic acid, in the blood, but as yet is not diagnosable ante-natally. Cystic fibrosis is the most common lethal genetic disorder among Caucasians, with 1 in 20 individuals being a carrier for this autosomal recessive disorder. As yet no ante-natal diagnosis is widely available although it has been achieved by specific assays on amniotic fluid supernatant.

50   B D E

The sex chromosome trisomy 47XXY is known as Klinefelter's syndrome. Mongolism, or Down's syndrome, is a trisomy of autosome 21. The Barr body represents the inactive X chromosome material adjacent to the nuclear membrane in normal female cells; in any genotype with more than one X chromosome the additional chromatin will be present as Barr bodies, one for each additional X; thus XXY individuals have 1 Barr body, XXXY 2 Barr bodies etc. Such individuals usually develop gynaecomastia at puberty, and are infertile, having under-developed testes. Older individuals are frequently mentally subnormal.

51   B D E

Toxoplasma gondii is the protozoan parasite responsible for toxoplasmosis. The life cycle of the parasite involves the domestic cat. The risk of contracting the illness in the UK is small (estimated as <0.2% in recent surveys) but higher in France (6%). Fetal involvement appears greater the earlier in pregnancy the infection occurs. The common fetal manifestations are growth retardation, hepatosplenomegaly, jaundice, anaemia, petechiae, retinopathy, hydrocephaly and convulsions. Choroido-retinitis and intracranial calcification may not develop for several months after birth.

52   E

Rubella virus is usually transmitted by droplet infection and has an incubation period of between 17-22 days. When infection occurs in adult life it is often subclinical and may go undiagnosed without serological testing. The fetal risks of infection reduce with advancing gestation, congenital malformations occurring in up to 50% of those infected in the first month but less than 20% of those occurring after the fourth month (sixteen weeks). Rubella specific IgM usually disappears a few weeks after the infection although it may occasionally persist for a year or more.

53 A B C
The vagina is sterile at birth but becomes rapidly colonised with Doderlein's bacilli (*Lactobacillus acidiphilus*) within 72 hours. This colonisation occurs because the vaginal mucosa of the newborn reflects the oestrogen status of late pregnancy and has a squamous epithelium many layers thick, the cells of which are rich in glycogen; within 2-3 weeks however, most of the superficial layers are exfoliated. Along with these epithelial changes the acid reaction of the newborn vagina becomes alkaline and remains so up to puberty. Thereafter again increasing oestrogen levels encourage glycogen formation within the superficial layers of the epithelium; this encourages recolonisation with lactobacilli, and the reaction becomes acid again. This has a protective effect against infection which is not possessed by the oestrogen deficient vagina of the pre-pubertal child or post-menopausal woman.

54 C D E
The Clostridia are anaerobic Gram-positive spore-forming bacilli. *Clostridium welchii (Cl. perfringens)* is the commonest of several members of the genus that may be associated with gas gangrene. Five types (A-E) may be differentiated by the exotoxins they produce, type A being that most commonly associated with gas gangrene. Infection with gas gangrene organisms may take 3 forms, firstly simple contamination, secondly spread along intramuscular septa, and thirdly invasion into healthy muscle by the exotoxin to produce a clostridial myonecrosis.

55 A B D
Proteus organisms are widely distributed in nature and are commonly found in the faeces of man and animals. Lactobacilli are normal commensals both in the vagina of women of reproductive age and in the bowel. Pneumococci are a normal inhabitant of the upper respiratory tract, although they are pathogenic in the lung, where they are associated with lobar pneumonia. *Streptococcus viridans* is a normal commensal of the mouth. The bladder is not colonised by bacteria under normal circumstances.

56 B C E
The internal iliac artery is a terminal branch of the common iliac artery. It has four visceral and seven parietal branches:

      Visceral   1.   Superior vesical a.
                  2.   Uterine a.
                  3.   Middle rectal a.

	4.	Vaginal a.
Parietal	1.	Umbilical a.
	2.	Obturator a.
	3.	Internal pudendal a.
	4.	Inferior gluteal a.
	5.	Superior gluteal a.
	6.	Lateral sacral a.
	7.	Iliolumbar a.

The anterior branch supplies all the visceral arteries and the first four parietal arteries. The posterior branch provides only the last three of the parietal branches and no visceral branches.

57   A B C

Lymph from the uterine tube drains along the ovarian artery to the para-aortic nodes. The corpus or body of the uterus drains mainly to the internal, external and common iliac nodes. Some channels pass along the round ligaments to the superficial inguinal nodes and others with the ovarian vessels to para-aortic nodes. Drainage of the cervix also includes the obturator nodes. The vagina drains in its upper two thirds to the internal and external iliac nodes and in the lower one third to the upper superficial inguinal nodes. The vulvar drainage of lymph is both ipsilateral and contralateral to the inguinal, internal iliac nodes and femoral nodes of the superficial and deep groups.

58   B C

The obturator nerve is formed within the psoas muscle from the anterior divisions of the 2nd, 3rd, and 4th lumbar nerves. It descends medial to psoas and runs along the lateral pelvic wall to the obturator groove through which it passes to reach the thigh; in the thigh it divides into anterior and posterior branches. The anterior division provides a sensory branch to the hip joint and a cutaneous branch to the medial side of the thigh. The posterior division supplies an articular branch to the knee joint and a muscular motor branch to obturator externus and adductor magnus. The anterior division has muscular branches to gracilis, adductor brevis and adductor longus.

59   B

The ureter is widest at its dilated upper end, the renal pelvis, which may contain a volume of 8 ml. The narrowest calibre is found at the pelvi-ureteric junction, where it crosses the pelvic brim and at its termination in the bladder mucosa. The ureter passes down the psoas muscle and crosses the genitofemoral nerve. It leaves the psoas muscle at the bifurcation of the common iliac artery, over the

119

sacroiliac joint and passes into the pelvis. The ureter then descends on the pelvic wall to the ischial spine before turning forwards and medially under the root of the broad ligament. Here it is crossed superiorly by the uterine artery and lies in close relation with the lateral fornix of the vagina just before entering the bladder. Blood supply is provided by a longitudinal anastomosis between the renal, ovarian, common iliac and inferior vesical arteries. Sympathetic nerve supply is derived from L1 to L3.

60 A C D
The ischio-rectal fossae are wedge-shaped spaces, the bases being inferior between the ischium and the anal canal. Supero-medially is levator ani attached to obturator fascia above and external anal sphincter below. Laterally the boundaries are fascial on obturator internus and inferiorly by perineal skin. The two fossae communicate with each other round the anal canal and are separated by the anococcygeal body, the anal canal and the perineal body, not by the vagina. The internal pudendal nerves and vessels lie in the lateral walls of the fossae within a sheath the pudendal canal. The fossae are filled with soft fat forming a dead space into which the anal canal can expand during defaecation.

ANSWERS TO PRACTICE EXAM 4

1 D E
Gluteus maximus, the prominent muscle of the buttock, is a powerful lateral rotator and extensor at the hip joint and acting through the iliotibial tract, it extends and stabilises the knee joint. It is supplied by the inferior gluteal nerve. Piriformis arises inside the pelvis from the anterior surface of the sacrum and passes laterally out of the greater sciatic foramen to be attached to the upper border of the greater trochanter of the femur. Psoas major arises from the five intervertebral discs above lumbar vertebrae and adjacent vertebral bodies and lumbar transverse processes; it is inserted into the lesser trochanter of the femur and flexes and medially rotates the femur at the hip. Psoas minor is a slender muscle lying on the surface of psoas major which arises from the intervertebral disc above the 1st lumbar vertebra and is attached to the arcuate line and iliopectineal eminence. Iliacus is attached to the upper two thirds of the hollow of the iliac fossa, it forms a common tendon with psoas attaching to the lesser trochanter and its function is therefore similar i.e. flexion and medial rotation.

2   **A B D E**
Laterally the anterior abdominal wall consists of three separate
sheet-like layers of muscle, an outer external oblique, an intermediate internal oblique and an inner transversalis abdominis.
Anteriorly they become aponeurotic, fuse and form the sheath
around the rectus abdominis. Above the umbilicus the internal
oblique aponeurosis splits to invest the rectus muscle and is re-
inforced anteriorly by the external oblique and posteriorly by the
transversus abdominis. External oblique originates from the outer
surfaces of the lower eight ribs. The superior epigastric artery and
the inferior epigastric artery with which it anastomoses both lie
deep to the rectus abdominis. The obliterated umbilical artery,
known in the adult as the lateral umbilical ligament passes obliquely
across the posterior wall of the inguinal canal, medial to the inferior
epigastric artery. The pyramidalis muscle arises from the pubic
crest between the rectus abdominis and its sheath and converges
with its fellow into the linea alba an inch or so above its origin; it is
frequently absent.

3   **C D E**
The cranial end of the paramesonephric duct in the female persists
and opens directly into the peritoneal cavity; it becomes the uterine
tube. The more caudal portions of the two ducts cross medial to the
mesonephric ducts and fuse together to form the definitive uterus
and upper vagina. Peritoneum covers the majority of the uterus
posteriorly as it covers the fundus, body and supravaginal part of
the cervix also passing onto the posterior wall of the vagina. The
uterus is supported and stabilised by the parametrial ligaments: the
uterosacrals, the lateral cervical or cardinal ligaments and pubocervical ligaments. The nerves of the uterus are branches from the
inferior hypogastric plexus. The uterus fails to acquire an
anteverted position in some 20% of women.

4   **B D E**
Meckel's diverticulum is a vestige of the vitello-intestinal duct
which may persist in 2-3% of the population. It is usually found on
the antemesenteric border of the ileum, within 75 cm of the ileo-
caecal junction. Its length may vary from little more than a dimple
on the bowel wall connected to the umbilicus by a fibrous band, to
being patent throughout its length, to communicate with the
umbilicus. It may contain gastric, colonic, hepatic, or pancreatic
tissues which may present with ulcerative symptoms.

5   **C D**
The vagina is lined by stratified squamous epithelium. Its anterior
and posterior walls (not the lateral walls) are normally in contact

except at its upper end into which projects the cervix surrounded by a deep sulcus, the fornix. At its upper end it projects above the pelvic floor into the peritoneal cavity. The upper part of the vagina is clasped by the pelvic floor fibres that loop around behind it. The U-shaped sling so formed is named the pubovaginalis (sphincter vaginae). A perineal sphincter (bulbospongiosus) surrounds its outlet. Vaginal lubrication is largely provided by mucus secreted by the cervix but also during sexual arousal by secretions from Bartholin's glands.

6 B D
As the femoral artery and vein pass beneath the inguinal ligament, they draw around themselves a funnel-shaped prolongation of the extraperitoneal fascia, transversalis fascia in front and fascia iliaca behind, known as the femoral sheath. The lacunar or Gimbernat's ligament lies medial to the sheath, and the femoral nerve lateral. The genito-femoral nerve is formed within the substance of psoas major from L1 and L2 roots; it divides into its genital and femoral branches above the inguinal ligament. The former pierces transversalis fascia to enter the spermatic cord, and the latter passes down in front of the femoral artery, piercing the femoral sheath to supply the skin of the thigh below the middle of the inguinal ligament.

7 A B
The female urethra is 3-5 cm in length; it is lined proximally by transitional epithelium continuous with the bladder, and distally by squamous epithelium continuous with the introital skin. The exact level of the squamo-transitional junction may vary, in particular with oestrogen status. The intrinsic urethral smooth muscle is orientated largely longitudinally or obliquely, and has little or no sphincteric activity. The intrinsic striated muscle (the rhabdosphincter urethrae) is maximal in bulk in mid-urethra anteriorly, thinning laterally and being almost totally deficient posteriorly. Its somatic supply from S2, 3 and 4, has recently been shown to travel in the nervi erigentes, although many traditional texts suggest it comes from the pudendal nerve.

8 A B E
The anal canal is closed by the internal (smooth muscle) and external (striated muscle) sphincters. The internal sphincter surrounds the upper 2/3 of the canal and is supplied by sympathetic and parasympathetic fibres from the pelvic plexus. The external sphincter surrounds the lower 2/3 of the canal and receives somatic supply from S3,4 via the inferior haemorrhoidal nerves and the perineal branch of S4. It is arranged in three distinct bundles, subcutaneous, superficial, and deep; at least some activity in the deep external

sphincter is necessary to maintain continence of faeces and flatus.

9   B E
The anterior primary rami of the upper four lumbar nerves form a plexus within the substance of psoas major; its branches are iliohypogastric (L1) ilioinguinal (L1), genitofemoral (L1-2), lateral cutaneous nerve of thigh (post divisions of L2-3), femoral (posterior divisions L2-4) and obturator (anterior divisions of L2-4). Much of L4 and all of L5 and the upper four sacral nerves form the sacral plexus on the front of pyriformis muscle. Several branches come from the main nerves before separation into anterior and posterior divisions. These include the pudendal, from S2-4 which supplies the pelvic floor and perineum, and the perineal branch of S4 which supplies the anal margin and part of the external anal sphincter.

10   A B D E
Insulin is anabolic, increasing the storage of glucose, fatty acids and amino acids. Insulin affects protein metabolism both by increasing the transport of amino acids into cells and also by stimulating nucleic acid synthesis. Lipogenesis and the esterification of fatty acids are stimulated by insulin and the rate of release of fatty acids is thereby reduced. The synthesis of long-chain fatty acids is facilitated by insulin. In liver and muscle, insulin increases the rate of glycogen formation and reduces the output of glucose. The activity of the enzyme glycogen synthetase is increased in muscle and liver as is liver glucokinase: gluconeogenesis and hepatic glycogenesis are inhibited. Infusions of insulin and glucose together significantly lower the plasma potassium levels and are effective for the temporary relief of hyperkalaemia in patients with renal failure.

11   B C D
The anterior pituitary or adenohypophysis develops as an ectodermal outgrowth from the roof of the pharynx, and thus contains no neural elements. The posterior part of the gland (neurohypophysis) is a downward extension from the diencephalon. The gland receives its blood supply from the superior and inferior hypophyseal branches of the internal carotid arteries; there is in addition a portal venous system connecting the hypothalamic neurosecretory centres with the anterior pituitary. Both FSH and LH are secreted by the basophil cells of the anterior pituitary. Oxytocin is secreted in the supraoptic and paraventricular nuclei of the hypothalamus and stored and released from the neurohypophysis.

12   A B D E

The effects of cortisol, whether endogenously produced or administered therapeutically, include:

— increased gluconeogenesis and peripheral antagonism to insulin thus causing hyperglycaemia
— a reduction in all components of the inflammatory response including reduced passage of fluid and cells out of capillaries and decreased fibrous tissue reaction
— eosinophil and lymphocyte counts are reduced whereas neutrophils red cells and platelets are increased.
— gastric acid and pepsin secretions are increased and may lead to peptic ulceration.

13   A B

95% of the cortisol entering the circulation is bound to protein, part to the α globulin transcortin, and part to albumin. The binding affinity of transcortin is much greater than that of albumin, but since the latter is present in much greater quantity, it carries a greater proportion of total cortisol. During pregnancy and after oestrogen administration, levels of transcortin rise; in cirrhosis and certain dysproteinaemias there is a reduction in cortisol binding power.

14   A B C E

During follicular development the first meiotic division, arrested in prophase during intrauterine development, is resumed about 36 hours prior to ovulation and is completed with the extrusion of the first polar body a few hours prior to ovulation. The second meiotic division proceeds as far as metaphase, to be completed only after fertilisation, which usually occurs in the ampullary region of the tube. The morula usually enters the uterus 3-5 days after fertilisation and shortly thereafter implantation occurs. Cervical mucus ferning, characteristic of oestrogen predominance, is usually lost within a short time after ovulation as progesterone secretion from the corpus luteum increases.

15   A C D

Ovarian activity in humans is cyclical, the production and release of oocytes by the ovary being episodic and coordinated with its endocrine activity. FSH is largely responsible for the growth of antral follicles to maturity. The LH surge causes changes in the follicle cells of the most advanced oocyte that result in the expulsion of the oocyte at ovulation. The period prior to ovulation is characterised by oestrogen dominance, after ovulation by progestogen and oestrogen together. Both the rise in basal body temperature and the disappearance of cervical mucus ferning are attributed to the progesterone produced by the corpus luteum which forms after oocyte expulsion. Anovulation is one cause of amenorrhoea but the relationship is not absolute. Conversely regular menstruation does not necessarily indicate regular ovulation.

16   A B C D
Coagulation factors I, VII, VIII, IX and X are all present in increased concentration in the plasma in normal pregnancy, from about the 3rd month of gestation. Plasma fibrinogen levels increase from a mean non-pregnant level of 2-4 g/l to 6 g/l in late pregnancy. Findings in relation to factors V, XI, XII and XIII are less consistent although if anything XII and XIII appear to decrease in concentration as pregnancy progresses.

17   A B D
Trophoblast cells may be found in the decidua basalis and myometrium and it has been estimated that up to 10,000 clumps of cells may be released daily into the maternal circulation to be lysed in the lung. It was at one time suggested that syncytiotrophoblast may be derived from granulosa cells of the ovary, but there is now no doubt that it is fetal in origin. The endometrium constitutes a partial immunologically privileged site because of its limited lymphatic supply; this privilege is important since the trophoblast is not immunologically inert, but expresses HLA antigens, albeit in low levels. Syncytiotrophoblast secretes HCG in addition to HPL, Schwangerschaft's protein (SP_1), various other pregnancy associated proteins, and steroids.

18   A B C
Fetal lung alveoli are lined by a group of phospholipids known collectively as 'surfactant', which prevent collapse of the alveoli during respiration by reducing surface tension. The predominant phospholipid is phosphatidyl choline (lecithin) and a surge in its production occurs at around 35 weeks gestation in normal pregnancy, promoted by glucocorticoids. Fetal lung maturity seems to be accelerated in some cases of pre-eclampsia, growth retardation, and premature rupture of the membranes and is delayed in diabetes mellitus. Alpha-fetoprotein is of no relevance to pulmonary maturity.

19   B C E
Angiotensin II levels are increased in normal pregnancy, although vascular sensitivity is reduced and it is unlikely that this factor is of relevance to altered uterine blood flow. The most significant factors are the increased blood volume and reduced uterine vascular resis-

tance resulting from dilatation of the arcuate arteries. The actual number of vessels does not change.

20   A C E

Human chorionic gonadotrophin (HCG) is produced by the placental trophoblast and some other tissues but not by fetal liver. The level in maternal serum rises rapidly in early pregnancy reaching a peak between 8 and 10 weeks of pregnancy. There is then a rapid reduction to 18 weeks after which levels remain more or less constant until delivery. HCG almost certainly rescues the corpus luteum from dissolution and promotes placental steroidogenesis. It is also important in the induction of fetal testosterone secretion by Leydig cells in the male fetus. It is suggested that HCG mediates the immunological privilege afforded to the fetus. A variety of gonadal and non-gonadal tumours have been reported to produce HCG; these include tumours of lung, stomach, liver, breast, kidney, pancreas, ovary and testis, carcinoid tumours and lymphomas.

21   A B D E

Inulin is freely filtered through the glomeruli and is neither secreted nor reabsorbed by the tubules and therefore can be used to measure glomerular filtration rate. GFR is influenced by three factors:- the size of the capillary bed, the permeability of the capillaries and the hydrostatic and osmotic pressure gradients across the capillary wall. As osmotic pressure of the filtrate in the tubule is negligible, this latter gradient is equal to the osmotic pressure of the plasma in the glomerular capillaries. At least 90% of filtered water is normally reabsorbed; the remainder of the filtered water can be reabsorbed without affecting total solute excretion. The descending limb of the loop of Henle is permeable to water but the ascending limb is relatively impermeable. Acid secretion by the tubular cells of the kidney is facilitated by carbonic anhydrase which catalyzes the reaction $CO_2 + H_2O = H_2CO_3$.

22   A B D E

Squamous cell carcinoma and adenocarcinoma of the cervix are equally sensitive to radiation. Dysgerminomas are noted for their predeliction to lymphatic spread and their acute sensitivity to irradiation. Carcinoma of the vulva would respond to radiotherapy in high doses but the effect on adjacent normal vulval skin would be so severe as to contraindicate this form of treatment.

23   A B D

Potassium is the principal cation in intracellular fluids. Deficiency, as manifest by hypokalaemia, causes muscle weakness (both somatic and visceral), mental confusion and interferes with neuromuscular transmission. The latter is evidenced by ECG changes e.g. depression of the ST segment, flattening or inversion of T-waves and prolongation of the PR interval. Hypokalaemia is associated with a reduced sensitivity of the renal tubules to ADH and the kidney therefore has a reduced concentrating ability, and frequency and polyuria are common symptoms. Since K^+ and H^+ compete for Na^+ exchange in the proximal convoluted tubule in K^+ depletion more H^+ will be lost in the urine, and a metabolic alkalosis result.

24   A B C D E
Formaldehyde produces BCME, a lung carcinogen in acid solution. Asbestos is known to predispose to tumours of lung, pleura and peritoneum. Chromium in paints and dyes has been implicated in lung cancer as has the nickel in welding alloys. Wood dust has been suggested to be a carcinogen to nasal sinuses.

25   E
The cytoplasm is pale and homogeneous in hydropic degeneration. The cytoplasm is eosinophilic in hyaline degeneration. Pyknosis refers to clumping of nuclear material and karyorrhexis to fragmentation of nuclear material and cell death.

26   A B D
The rates of some enzyme catalysed reactions are increased in the presence of certain ions which do not themselves appear in the overall reaction equation, these are called activators (e.g. carbonic anhydrase requires Zn^{2+} for its activity). Coenzymes are organic compounds essential to the activity of some enzymes, not firmly bound to their enzymes but freely dissociable. Prosthetic groups on the other hand are non-amino acid groups which are relatively firmly bound to a protein 'apo-enzyme' but which again play an important catalytic role. All of these factors can be recycled over and over in the same reaction or group of reactions since they are unchanged by the metabolic processes involved. This is in distinction to the enzyme substrate which is irreversibly altered at the end of the reaction. Many of the substances acting as B group vitamins in the human diet e.g. nicotinamide, riboflavin, thiamin, biotin, pantothenic acid, folic acid, cobalamin, and pyridoxal are chemically related to coenzymes or prothetic groups. They cannot be synthesised, at least not in adequate quantities, and are essential dietary requirements.

27   A B E
Cervix uteri, gall bladder and bronchus all contain squamous epithelium which may undergo metaplasia; liver and stomach do not.

28 D E

When there is obstruction to the flow of bile, either intra- or extra-hepatically, the process of conjugation of bilirubin by the hepatocytes will initially proceed normally. Conjugated bilirubin, therefore, no longer excreted via the bile ducts, accumulates in the plasma. This is a relatively small molecule, since it is not protein bound and is therefore readily excreted in urine. Since the flow of conjugated bilirubin down the bile duct is interrupted, the production of stercobilinogen by intestinal bacteria is reduced, and this along with its oxidation product stercobilin is present in reduced amounts in faeces. The reabsorption and enterohepatic circulation of these pigments is also therefore reduced and their excretion in urine as urobilinogen and urobilin decreases.

It is not clear how plasma alkaline phosphatase levels relate to hepatic excretory function but their determination is of value in the jaundiced patient. In post-hepatic (obstructive) jaundice, levels rise markedly; in hepatitic jaundice the elevation is usually of lesser degree, and in pre-hepatic (haemolytic) jaundice levels usually remain normal.

29 A D E

Sarcoidosis is a systemic disease of uncertain aetiology, characterised histologically by epithelioid cells in a discrete follicle. Schaumann bodies refer to spherical basophilic masses in Langhan's giant cells, which may be found amongst the epithelioid cells. Unlike the tubercle follicle, there is never any true caseation and no round cell infiltration.

30 A C

Local invasion or distant metastases to regional lymph nodes are characteristic features of malignancy. Pleomorphism which is the marked difference in size, shape and other morphological features of cells is seen in dysplastic or anaplastic cells and is therefore more likely to indicate malignancy. An intact capsule and well differentiated histology are common features of benign tumours.

31 B C D

Metaplasia is the transformation of one type of tissue into another; as such it usually represents a response to a call for altered function or is the result of an altered environment. This process is in marked contrast to anaplasia which represents the reversion of a more highly to a less highly differentiated tissue. Metaplasia is not a form of in situ malignant change. Squamous metaplasia may occur in the bladder or endometrium especially in response to changes in oestrogen status, and in the cervix, when the endocervical glandular epithelium becomes exposed to the low pH of the vagina.

32   B D
During pregnancy, thyroid hormone binding globulin levels increase in the first trimester under the influence of oestrogen; T3 and T4 production are increased but the free levels of these hormones are unchanged. Neither TSH nor thyroid hormones themselves cross the placenta to any significant extent.

The developing thyroid is first recognised as a thickening on the floor of the pharynx at around 4 weeks gestation; it does not begin to function however until the end of the 1st trimester. Fetal TSH production begins at around the same time and levels increase steadily between 20 and 30 weeks gestation, increasing further after delivery, but usually returning to normal adult levels within 3 days. In cretinism the deficiency of thyroid hormone leads to a persistently elevated TSH level.

33   A B D
Human placental lactogen is not detectable in the non-pregnant female but can be detected from 5 weeks gestation, its concentration increasing with advancing gestation to around 35 weeks. The shape of the concentration curve closely resembles that of placental growth and levels tend to be increased in situations associated with increased placental weight e.g. multiple pregnancy. It has both growth hormone and prolactin like properties and among its metabolic effects are an increase in plasma free fatty acids due to maternal fat mobilisation and an increased insulin resistance causing higher circulating insulin and an increased insulin response to a glucose load.

34   A C E
Cyproterone acetate is a 17-alpha-methyl-beta-testosterone which acts as an anti-androgen at the hair follicle level, competing with testosterone for receptors; it also decreases gonadotrophin production centrally. It is used in the treatment of hirsutism and virilism usually combined with an oestrogen preparation. It tends to suppress ovulation. The safety of cyproterone in pregnancy has not been demonstrated; it is known to cause feminisation of the fetus in rats.

35   B D E
Follicle stimulating hormone (FSH) is secreted by the basophil cells of the anterior pituitary, release being governed by gonadal steroids acting at a hypothalamic level modulating the production of

gonadotrophin releasing hormone and also directly on the pituitary. Oestrogen has both negative and positive feedback effects and alters the proportion of LH and FSH secreted in response to GnRH. Low oestrogen status e.g. in the post-menopausal woman, in Turner's syndrome, and in pure gonadal dysgenesis are all characterised by grossly elevated FSH levels. In Sheehan's syndrome, pan-hypopituitarism resulting from post partum hypoxic pituitary necrosis, FSH levels are inevitably low. Combined oestrogen-progesterone contraceptive pills inhibit ovulation by interference with feedback mechanisms at the hypothalamic level.

36 C D

Cortisol is produced from the zona fasiculata of the adrenal cortex; the zona glomerulosa secretes aldosterone. There is a diurnal rhythm of ACTH secretion initiated by the hypothalamus which leads to variation in cortisol output, levels being maximal between 6 and 8 am and lowest at midnight. Production of cortisol is increased in response to hypoglycaemia. This results in an increase in gluconeogenesis, peripheral antagonism to insulin, and normo- or hyperglycaemia.

The substances assayed in the urine as 17 oxogenic steroids are essentially derived from the 17 hydroxycorticosteroids cortisol, cortisone, and their tetrahydro derivatives.

The obesity of Cushing's syndrome is typically truncal, being maximal on the face, supraclavicular fossae and over the 7th cervical vertebra, the limbs being relatively spared.

37 D E

ACTH appears to act on specific surface receptors on the adrenocortical cell membranes and alters cortisol secretion via the cyclic AMP system. Aldosterone is normally produced in response to changes in the renin-angiotensin system. Renin is secreted from the juxta-glomerular cells in the kidney; this acts on the α_2 globulin angiotensinogen to produce the decapeptide angiotensin I. A pulmonary converting enzyme yields the octopeptide angiotensin II which is a powerful vasopressor agent as well as a stimulator of aldosterone release. Renin release may be stimulated by decreased renal perfusion, or extracellular fluid volume e.g. from hypotension or dehydration or by sodium depletion. ACTH has a 'permissive effect' on zona glomerulosa by ensuring adequate steroid precursors for aldosterone production. The major effects of aldosterone are to decrease urinary sodium and water excretion with increased potassium losses; the typical biochemical findings in primary

hyperaldosteronism therefore are hypokalaemia and hypernatraemia.

38 A B D E
Histamine is a vasoactive substance, particularly important in the
early stages of acute inflammation. It causes contraction of
extravascular smooth muscle, dilatation of blood vessels and
increases capillary permeability. 5-hydroxytryptamine, or serotonin, is released from mast cells and plays a similar role to
histamine. Bradykinin causes smooth muscle contraction but more
slowly than histamine. It also vasodilates and is the most powerful
active permeability factor known, in addition to producing pain.
Prostacyclin, (PGI$_2$) which is produced by the endothelial cells of
blood vessels, causes vasodilation and increases permeability.
Angiotensin reduces capillary permeability.

39 C D E
Cephaloridine should only be given intramuscularly or
intravenously because of poor absorption when taken orally. Renal
toxicity occurs with high doses and in those with reduced renal
function; toxicity is enhanced by diuretics. Cephalosporins are
related to the penicillins in that both contain a ß-lactam ring. This
gives the cephalosporins a similar mode of action and a spectrum
similar to ampicillin; also there is partial cross-allergenicity.

40 A C E
Beta-adrenergic blocking agents can cause neonatal hypoglycaemia
and interfere with maternal diabetic control. The drugs are con-
strictors of bronchial smooth muscle and so will exacerbate asthma.
They should also be avoided in heartblock as they cause bradycardia, encourage sodium retention and aggravate heart failure. Their
action in reducing blood pressure is produced by lowering cardiac
output; peripheral vascular resistance tends to rise. Patients with
symptomatic hyperthyroidism may have enhanced sympathetic
activity and increased responsiveness to beta adrenergic stimulation; beta adrenergic blocking agents are used when these features
are severe.

41 B C
Glucocorticoids, of which hydrocortisone (cortisol) is one,
decrease the number of circulating eosinophils by increasing their
sequestration in the spleen and lungs. They increase protein
catabolism and increase hepatic glycogenesis and gluconeogenesis.
Glucose-6-phosphatase activity is increased and the blood glucose
rises. In excessive amounts such as is seen in Cushing's syndrome
glucocorticoids lead to bone dissolution, elevated glomerular filtra-

tion rate and increased calcium excretion. In addition significant K^+ depletion may result from increased excretion.

42 A B C

Bromocryptine is a semisynthetic ergot alkaloid. It is rapidly and extensively absorbed from the gastrointestinal tract. Its peak plasma concentration occurs 2-3 hours following ingestion. A single dose is able to suppress prolactin levels within 3-4 hours and its action will continue for 8-12 hours. Bromocryptine is a dopamine agonist, believed to act directly on the dopamine receptors in the prolactin secreting cells of the pituitary gland. It is a vasoconstrictor and therefore should not be used in patients with coronary vascular or peripheral vascular disease. Bromocryptine has been widely used in the treatment of infertility and there is no evidence that it is teratogenic.

43 A E

Average testosterone levels in the male are ten times higher than in the female and the normal ranges are quite separate. In the premenopausal woman 50% of circulating testosterone is derived from the conversion of ovarian (20%) and adrenal (30%) androstenedione, this being the main androgen produced by the ovaries, and the interconversion readily achieved by the enzyme 17β hydroxysteroid dehydrogenase. Only 30% of circulating testosterone is actually secreted as such by the adrenal, but dehydroepiandrosterone is produced almost exclusively by the adrenals.

44 C

Transient immunity to some infections can be achieved by passive transfer of appropriate antibodies by injection of serum from an immune individual or animal. Rubella is the only one of the above listed diseases in which passive immunity is employed. It is effective only if given before exposure and efficacy is doubtful. Specific antibodies cannot be raised against the antigens of the others.

45 C

Formalin inactivates the toxigenicity of proteinaceous bacterial endotoxins without affecting their immunogenicity. Toxins detoxified in this manner are referred to as toxoids. Toxoids prepared from the toxins of *Corynebacterium diphtheriae* (diphtheria toxoid) and *Clostridium tetani* (tetanus toxoid) are used routinely in immunisation schedules. It retains its immunogenicity and so can be phagocytosed, can stimulate an immune response and gives a precipitin reaction with antibody.

46   B D E

The clinical effects of bacteraemic shock result from absorbed endotoxins usually from Gram-negative organisms including *Escherichia coli*, *Bacillus proteus* and *Klebsiella aerogenes*. Toxic damage to blood vessel walls leads to a loss of circulating fluid and protein into the extravascular space, and a leukopaenia is commonly seen. Massive doses of steroids may be helpful in reducing the passage of fluid and cells across capillary walls and also by sensitising arterioles to the effects of circulating noradrenaline and thereby maintaining blood pressure.

47   A B C D E

Coxsackie B virus infection, associated with Borholm disease, but often unrecognised in the mother may be transmitted to the fetus and give rise to a myocarditis or meningoencephalitis in the neonate; it has also been implicated as a possible cause of structural congenital heart and urogenital abnormalities.

Cytomegalovirus also is often asymptomatic in the mother and may be transmitted to the fetus or neonate transplacentally, or during passage through the birth canal, or during breast feeding. Infection in pregnancy may be associated with increased rate of abortion or premature delivery. Those infants born alive may be of low birth weight and may suffer fulminating disease in the neonatal period, with jaundice thrombocytopenic purpura, and choroidoretinitis. Chronic infection may be associated with spasticity, microcephaly and mental retardation.

Hepatitis B may be transmitted transplacentally and is associated with neonatal hepatitis.

Pregnant women show an increased susceptibility, severity, and mortality from poliomyelitis; the fetus may be infected leading to intrauterine fetal death or neonatal paralysis.

Transplacental passage of herpes virus type 2 is uncommon although the infant may become infected during passage through the birth canal and develop a fatal disseminated infection.

48   B D E

Ascorbic acid is a water-soluble vitamin found in citrus fruits and green vegetables; milk and meat contain only traces. Vitamin C is easily destroyed by oxidation at moderate temperatures; consequently large losses occur in cooking. Freezing of food does not disrupt vitamin C. The vitamin serves a vital role in collagen synthesis and wound healing.

49   A D E

Krebs cycle is also called the citric acid cycle and produces by oxidation metabolic energy in the form of ATP. It is the process responsible for harnessing the contained chemical energy in carbohydrates, but it is not purely catabolic, facilitating as it does the synthesis of essential metabolites such as amino acids and long chain fatty acids. The cycle depends upon a continuous supply of oxidised co-enzyme for its maintenance and does allow the complete combustion of fatty acids.

50   A B D

Vitamin B_{12} is produced by moulds and fungi but is absent from all other plant products; the main dietary sources are liver, meat, eggs and milk. Like other B vitamins it is water soluble and is not destroyed by cooking. Daily requirements are quite low (1-3μg/day) and this is met by all but the most strictly vegetarian diets. Deficiency is characterised by a macrocytic megaloblastic anaemia and this is usually due to impaired absorption rather than dietary deficiency. Absorption of B_{12} occurs in the ileum and is dependent on the presence of 'intrinsic factor', a glycoprotein produced by the gastric mucosa. In true Addisonian pernicious anaemia or in gastrectomised patients the deficiency of intrinsic factor must be circumvented by parenteral administration of B_{12}

51   All false

The fetal gut is described in three regions, the foregut being that part supplied by the coeliac artery and lying proximal to the entry of the bile ducts, the hindgut supplied by the inferior mesenteric artery and lying distal to the splenic flexure and the midgut between, supplied by the superior mesenteric artery.

As the fetal midgut elongates at around 7 weeks gestation it forms a U-shaped loop, attached to the vitello-intestinal duct at its apex, which projects out through the abdominal wall into the umbilical cord.

This so-called herniation is necessary because of the paucity of space within the abdominal cavity and the relatively large size of the fetal liver and kidneys at this stage. By the 12th week the available space is relatively increased and the intestine returns rapidly to the abdominal cavity. In doing so it undergoes rotation in an anticlockwise direction around the axis of the superior mesenteric artery to bring the caudal limb of the loop, which will ultimately give rise to the caecum, to the right side of the abdomen.

52   C
The Mullerian or paramesonephric ducts develop lateral to the
Wolffian or mesonephric ducts as an invagination of the coelomic
epithelium overlying the nephrogenic ridge, at 5-6 weeks
embryonic development. The lower end of each Mullerian duct
fuses with a thickening on the posterior aspect of the urogenital
sinus known as the sinovaginal bulb. Their junctions form the
vaginal plate, a solid core of epithelium which becomes canalised at
16-18 weeks. The Mullerian ducts themselves fuse in their lower
part to form the uterovaginal primordium by 12 weeks, although
the cranial portions of the ducts remain separate and ultimately give
rise to the Fallopian tubes.

53   D
Alleles are alternative forms of a gene that may occupy the same
locus; any one chromosome bears only a single allele at any given
locus, although in the population as a whole there may be multiple
alleles, dominant or recessive, any one of which may occupy that
locus. They are thus complete genes, not parts of a gene or products
of a gene.

54   A B C D
Lymphoid stem cells may first be detected in the yolk sac, later in
the fetal liver, and subsequently in the bone marrow. They subsequently may mature within the bone marrow (B cells) or migrate
to the thymus (T cells) where they populate the area around the
periphery of the thymic cortex. T cells are responsible for cell
mediated immunity whereas the B cells are responsible for humoral
or antibody mediated immunity. T lymphocytes comprise around
70% of the 'recirculating pool' of lymphocytes in peripheral blood
and lymph nodes whereas B lymphocytes predominate in the marrow and spleen.

55   A
All we can conclude is that in some (unspecified) respect drug X was
discovered to be more effective than drug Y to an extent which one
would only expect to have arisen by chance in less than 1% of
occasions. The 'p' (probability) value tells us nothing about the type
of study, the number of patients investigated, the statistical test
performed or the prognosis for any individual patient as regards
improvement or side effects. (Indeed it is quite possible from the
data presented that the effectiveness may be very slight and side
effects considerable!)

56   A C
The endocervix has a secretory columnar epithelium which is main-

135

tained during menstruation. It is arranged in branched glands whose secretion is scanty and viscid early in the follicular phase, becomes profuse and clear under the influence of oestrogen towards ovulation and then becomes thick, opaque, and highly cellular with progesterone secretion in the luteal phase of the cycle. The corpus uteri has a largely muscular structure, the cervix a much larger fibrous content.

57 A B D
The inguinal (Poupart's) ligament extends from the anterior superior iliac spine to the pubic tubercle and is the free lower border of the external oblique aponeurosis. It is rolled inwards inferiorly into a gutter which forms the floor of the inguinal canal, from the deep to superficial inguinal rings. The ilio-inguinal nerve in the abdomen lies in the neurovascular plane between transversus abdominis and the internal oblique. It pierces the lower fibres of internal oblique to emerge on the spermatic cord to pass through the superficial ring; it thus lies above the ligament.

58 D E
The trigone is that area of the bladder base bounded by the two ureteric orifices and the internal urethral orifice. Being relatively fixed at these points it is the least mobile part of the bladder, and its appearance changes little with varying degrees of bladder distension. Its superficial muscle fibres are of relatively small diameter, giving it a smooth appearance on endoscopy compared to the often ridged or trabeculated appearance of the rest of the wall. Whilst the remainder of the bladder and urethra are formed from urogenital sinus the trigone is formed by the incorporation of the lower end of the mesonephric ducts into the bladder base. Sensation in the lower urinary tract is difficult to quantify although it seems that sensation in the urethra is considerably more acute than elsewhere.

59 A B D E
The typical female pelvic shape in the UK has a brim which is slightly wider in its transverse than A - P diameter (gynaecoid), the true obstetric conjugate being 11-12 cm and the transverse 13 cm. The cavity has the contours of a curved cylinder rather than a funnel, the side walls being approximately parallel. The greater sciatic notch is usually greater than 90° and the subpubic angle should also approximate to a right angle.

60 A D E
The femoral sheath is an investment of extraperitoneal fascia extending over the femoral artery and vein as they pass beneath the inguinal ligament; the vein lies medial to the artery in the sheath but

medial to the vein lies a space, the femoral canal. Lymph vessels from the deep inguinal nodes pass through this space which also contains the node of Cloquet. The canal is widest at its proximal end where its opening is known as the femoral ring; this is bounded anteriorly by the inguinal ligament, medially by the lacunar ligament, and laterally by the femoral vein. The femoral branch of the genito-femoral nerve passes in front of the femoral artery to pierce the femoral sheath and fascia lata, and thus lies well lateral to the femoral canal.

ANSWERS TO PRACTICE EXAM 5

1   A E

The ovarian artery on each side is a branch of the abdominal aorta just below the level of the renal arteries. The ovarian veins form a plexus in the mesovarium and infundibulo-pelvic ligament; a pair of veins on each side usually combine into a single trunk before their termination; that on the right joins the inferior vena cava and that on the left the left renal vein (this is embryologically symmetrical since on each side the vein concerned is a persistent part of the subcardinal vein of the embryo). The ovary is covered by a single layered cuboidal epithelium, the so-called germinal epithelium; it is attached to the posterior aspect of the broad ligament. The suspensory ligament of ovary connects the medial pole of the ovary to the uterine fundus — being part of the gubernaculum.

2   C D

The vagina develops in part from the paramesonephric or Mullerian ducts and in part from the urogenital sinus; the relative proportions of these two contributions are argued. The epithelium of the vagina is a non-keratinizing stratified squamous epithelium. The posterior relations of the vagina are the pouch of Douglas in the upper third, the rectum in the middle third and the perineal body in the lower third. The vaginal blood supply is from descending branches of the uterine arteries (upper third), lateral continuations of the inferior vesical arteries and terminal branches of the internal iliac arteries (middle third) and from ascending clitoral arteries (lower third).

3   A B D E

The ureter passes down the posterior abdominal wall on the psoas major muscle, being closely adherent to the overlying peritoneum. It passes over the genitofemoral nerve and enters the pelvis approximately at its midpoint, crossing the bifurcation of the common iliac artery. The ureter obtains its blood supply sequentially

137

from branches of the renal arteries, the aorta, the gonadal arteries, the common and internal iliac arteries, and the superior and inferior vesical arteries. It may course very close to the infundibulo-pelvic ligament, and this is one of the common sites of surgical injury to the ureter.

4   B E
The pudendal nerve arises from the anterior surfaces of the S2,3 and 4 nerve roots, whereas the nerve to obturator internus arises from the L5 and S1 and S2 roots. The pudendal nerve itself passes back between the pyriformis and coccygeus muscles to appear in the buttock between pyriformis and the sacrospinal ligament; thereafter it curves around the latter to run in the pudendal canal on the lateral wall of the ischio-rectal fossa. The inferior haemorrhoidal branch of the pudendal nerve supplies the subcutaneous and profundus portions of the external anal sphincter; the internal sphincter, however receives autonomic supply from the pelvic plexus. Cutaneous branches of the pundendal nerve supply the clitoris (from the dorsal nerve of clitoris) the labia majora and minora (from the perineal branch) and the perianal skin (from the inferior haemorrhoidal branch).

5   A B C D
The Fallopian tubes develop from the unfused rostral portions of the paramesonephric or Mullerian ducts. The calibre of the tube varies along its length being maximal in the ampullary region and minimal in the isthmus. The fimbria ovarica attaches the tube to the lateral pole of the ovary and presumably aids ovum transport into the tube following ovulation. The tubal lining is a single layered columnar epithelium containing ciliated secretory, and resting or peg cells; the secretory cells develop microvilli and become secretory at midcycle and ciliary activity also increases at ovulation.

6   All false
The uterine wall varies from 1-1.5 cm thick and the bulk of this thickness is composed of smooth muscle fibres of the myometrium. The isthmus is that portion of the uterus lying between the anatomical and histological internal os; whilst this region expands in midpregnancy it can be identified from puberty onwards. The uterus is maintained in position partly by the pelvic floor muscles but largely by ligaments, the cardinal (transverse cervical) ligaments laterally, the uterosacral ligaments posteriorly and the pubocervical ligaments anteriorly; the round ligaments play little part in normal uterine support. The blood supply to the uterus is largely from the uterine arteries although there is an anastomosis with a tubal branch of the ovarian arteries which contributes to the

supply of the uterine fundus. The nerve supply to the uterus comes from the pelvic plexus, sympathetic efferent supply from T_{12}-L_2 and visceral afferents from corpus to $T_{11,12}$ and L_1, and cervix to $S_{2,3}$ and 4.

7   **A B D E**
The broad ligament is a double-layered fold of peritoneum lying on either side of the uterus; its medial edge is continuous with the serosa overlying the uterus, and its lateral edge is attached to the pelvic side wall. The Fallopian tube lies in the medial three quarters of its upper edge, and the ovarian vessels in the lateral quarter of its upper edge. The ovary lies on the posterior surface of the broad ligament, its medial pole being attached to the cornu of the uterus by the ovarian ligament. The pelvic ureter passes forwards in the base of the broad ligament to enter obliquely into the base of the bladder. Apart from the structures already mentioned, the broad ligament contains a mass of areolar tissue, the uterine blood vessels and lymphatics and vestigeal remnants of the mesonephric (Wolffian) ducts, the epoophorn and the paroophorn.

8   **B D E**
The pelvic floor consists of a gutter-shaped sheet of striated muscle slung around the midline body effluents, the urethra, vagina, and anal canal. Although functioning as a unit, it consists morphologically of three muscles, the ischiococcygeus ('coccygeus' muscle), the iliococcygeus and the pubococcygeus (together known as the levator ani), from behind forward, taking origin in turn from the ischial spine, the arcus tendineus, and the posterior surface of the pubis. Anterior fibres of the pubococcygeus form a sling around the ano-rectal junction, joining with fibres from the opposite side and with posterior fibres of the profundus part of the external sphincter. Apart from the sphincteric functions of the muscles they also help to maintain the position of the pelvic organs, and to direct the internal rotation of the presenting part during labour. The nerve supply to the muscles is by the perineal branch of S_4, the inferior haemorrhoidal and perineal nerves, from the sacral plexus.

9   **A D**
The breast is an ectodermal structure developing from a downward growth of epidermis into the underlying mesenchyme, in a similar manner to which sweat glands develop, but occurring specifically along two thickened strips of ectoderm, the mammary ridges. Branching epithelial cords appear, become canalised in midgestation, and further proliferation and branching occurs up to full term and again at puberty. Lobular organisation within the breast occurs at puberty with the development ultimately of 15-20 lobes each of

which drains into a single lactiferous duct which opens via the lactiferous sinus onto the surface of the nipple; true secretory alveoli do not appear until the woman herself becomes pregnant. Although the mature breast varies greatly in size, its base is fairly constant extending from the 2nd to 6th ribs in the midclavicular line, and overlying pectoralis major, serratus anterior, and external oblique. The lymphatic drainage of the superficial parts of the breast is into a subareolar plexus, and of the deep parts into a submammary plexus, which communicate freely with each other, and with the opposite side. From these plexi lymph drains laterally to the pectoral group of axillary glands, superiorly to the infraclavicular glands, medially to the internal mammary and mediastinal glands, and inferiorly via lymph glands in the anterior abdominal wall through the diaphragm and on to the mediastinal glands.

10   A B D E
Cardiac output is the output of the heart per unit time. It is calculated by the product of the stroke volume and heart rate in beats per minute. The stroke volume is the amount of blood pumped out of each ventricle per beat. In the resting person in the supine position the stroke volume will average 80 ml (the actual volume put out by the two ventricles in series will be twice the stroke volume i.e. 80 ml from the left ventricle and 80 ml from the right). The cardiac output will usually increase when the heart rate increases but this is not true of rapid arrhythmias. Normal cardiac output will decrease on sitting or standing from the supine position and conversely will increase when the subject becomes supine after standing. A high environmental temperature will cause increased cardiac output via increased venous return

11   A C D
Deoxycorticosterone and aldosterone elevate the blood pressure and hypertension is a prominent feature of primary hyperaldosteronism. Hypertension is also seen in Cushing's syndrome in which aldosterone secretion is usually normal. Although the cause in this syndrome is uncertain it may be that increased circulating ACTH adrenocorticotrophic hormone produces an increase in secretion of deoxycorticosterone. Hypertension is usually due to increased peripheral resistance which is likely to cause left ventricular hypertrophy rather than the converse. Chronic respiratory failure leads to pulmonary vasoconstriction and pulmonary hypertension but is unlikely to affect systemic blood pressure unless severe polycythaemia is produced. Alpha-methyl dopa is a drug that depresses sympathetic activity by forming a false transmitter and therefore causes peripheral vasodilatation and hypotension.

12   A B E
Total cerebral blood flow is generally maintained at a constant level under varying conditions. Although there are significant shifts in the pattern of flow, total cerebral flow is not increased by strenuous mental activity. Mean arterial pressure does affect total cerebral blood flow positively. Changes in blood gas tensions affect cerebral arterioles; a low pO_2 is associated with vasodilatation while a rise in pCO_2 (hypercapnia) also exerts a potent dilator effect. Although cerebral vessels are innervated by noradrenergic vasoconstrictor fibres and cholinergic vasodilator fibres, vasomotor reflexes appear to play little if any part in the regulation of cerebral blood flow in humans.

13   A C D E
Carbon dioxide is transported in the blood, both in physical solution (5%) and in combined forms with haemoglobin, plasma proteins or bicarbonate (95%). The carbon dioxide that diffuses into red blood cells is rapidly hydrated to H_2CO_3 because of the presence of carbonic anhydrase. The H_2CO_3 dissociates to H^+ and HCO_3^-, the H^+ being buffered by haemoglobin. Since the HCO_3^- content of red cells is much greater than that of plasma, cell membranes being relatively impermeable to cation, much (around 70%) of the HCO_3^- diffuses out into the plasma, electrochemical neutrality is maintained by diffusion of Cl^- into the red cells (the so-called 'chloride shift'); CO_2 is not however transported as HCl in the blood. Some of the CO_2 in red cells reacts with the amino groups of proteins to form carbamino compounds. In the plasma CO_2 also reacts with plasma proteins to form small amounts of carbamino compounds, and small amounts are hydrated to H_2CO_3; this latter reaction is however slow in the absence of carbonic anhydrase. Most of the CO_2 in the plasma therefore is as bicarbonate whereas in erythrocytes the majority is as carbamino-haemoglobin.

14   A B C D E
Automatic spontaneous respiration is dependent upon nerve impulses from the pons and medulla causing discharge of motor neurones that innervate the respiratory muscles. This rhythmic discharge is modified by centres in the pons and by afferents in the vagus nerves arising from receptors in the lung parenchyma; stretching of the lungs during inspiration inhibits respiratory drive. An increase in pCO_2 or H^+ concentration or a decrease in pO_2 acts via chemoreceptors in the medulla, carotid and aortic bodies to stimulate respiratory centre activity. Inhibition of respiration and closure of the glottis prevent aspiration during swallowing, gagging and vomiting.

15   **A B D**
Normal erythropoiesis is dependent on adequate supplies of:

Amino acids —   for the synthesis of the globin component of haemoglobin and the red cell stroma.

Iron —   which is essential for the formation of haem prosthetic groups.

Vitamin B_{12} —   is necessary in nucleic acid synthesis in particular for the syntheses of labile methyl groups from one carbon precursors.

Folic acid —   is also necessary in nucleic acid synthesis for the movement of methyl groups from one acceptor to another.

Vitamin B_6 —   appears to function as a co-enzyme in the formation of haem.

Nicotinic acid (niacin) forms part of the co-enzymes NAD and NADP which act as hydrogen acceptors in oxidation reactions involving the flavoprotein cytochrome systems occurring in mitochondria. Myoglobin is an oxygen binding pigment found in muscle cells. Haem forms part of the structure of both myoglobin and cytochromes but neither are of relevance to erythropoiesis.

16   **A B**
The blood flow in the renal cortex is much greater than in the medulla and is grossly in excess of the metabolic needs of the kidneys. It is largely unrelated to arterial pressure and is able to alter renal vascular resistance to maintain renal blood flow at a fairly constant level. Renal blood flow is reduced by fear and emotional stress due to constriction of renal blood vessels but is unchanged by noradrenaline administration.

17   **A**
The glomerular filtration rate can be estimated by measuring the secretion and plasma level of a substance which is freely filtered through the glomeruli and neither secreted nor reabsorbed by the tubules. Inulin is a polymer of fructose which most closely approaches the above criteria and is used extensively to measure glomerular filtration. Insulin is largely metabolised and degraded in the kidneys and therefore unsuitable. Glucose is freely filtered but reabsorbed almost totally in the first part of the proximal tubule so is inappropriate. Glucagon has a very short half life in the circulation of 5-10 minutes due to liver degradation. Paraaminohippuric acid (PAH) is filtered by the glomeruli and secreted by the tubular cells and is used to measure effective renal plasma flow rather than GFR.

18   A B E

Micturition is dependent on a spinal reflex arc mediated via parasympathetic efferents and accompanying viseral afferent fibres synapsing within the conus medullaris at spinal level S2-4. Normal coordinated micturition is of course also dependent on higher central control involving additional relay centres in the pontine reticular formation (for the coordination of detrusor contraction with urethral relaxation), the basal ganglion (for subconscious inhibition of micturition) and in the paracentral lobule and superior frontal gyrus of the cerebral cortex (for the appreciation of the desire to void, conscious inhibition and then subsequent voluntary initiation of voiding). It is these latter cortical centres which give the detrusor its property, unique among smooth muscles, of being under voluntary control. Any neurological lesion below the pontine centre will lead to a discoordinate voiding pattern, with urethral contraction accompanying detrusor contraction, and thus a residual volume is likely to remain after voiding.

The lower urinary tract has a sympathetic nerve supply from spinal segments T_{12} - L_2; this seems to be of greater relevance to the filling and storage phases of the micturition cycle than to voiding itself, and transection of these fibres has little influence on micturition.

19   A C D E

Severe diarrhoea is extremely debilitating, and can be fatal especially in infants. Large quantities of sodium and potassium are washed out of the colon and small intestine in the diarrhoeal stools, leading to dehydration, hypovolaemia and ultimately to shock and cardiovascular collapse. Hypokalaemia may be particularly profound because of the high intra-lumenal concentrations of potassium in the ileum and colon.

20   C D

In the normal pregnant woman at rest, but not lying supine, cardiac output rises from early pregnancy to a peak at around 20 weeks gestation which is approximately 1.5 litres per minute, or 40% above the non-pregnant level; this rise is maintained through the rest of pregnancy. This increase in cardiac output is achieved both by an increase in heart rate (averaging 15 beats per minute) and stroke volume (from 65 to 70 ml); again these changes are present from early pregnancy. The general pattern in blood pressure seen by most observers suggests relatively little change in systolic pressure, but a marked fall in diastolic pressure which is lowest in midpregnancy and thereafter rises to approximate to non-pregnant levels again by term; for most of pregnancy therefore there is an increase in pulse pressure. Plasma volume changes vary with age, parity, race, and 'reproductive performance'. In healthy women in their first pregnancy plasma volume increases by about 40% over the non-pregnant level of 2600 ml, between 12 and 32 weeks gestation.

21   A B C E
The end result of blood coagulation is the formation of an insoluble fibrin clot from the soluble precursor fibrinogen in the plasma. The process involves a complex interaction of clotting factors and a sequential activation of a series of proenzymes each of which is assigned a Roman numeral I - XII; fibrinogen is designated coagulation factor I; calcium functions as a metal activator in several of the cascade reactions and is designated factor IV. Heparin is a naturally occurring anticoagulant found in mast cells, which potentiates the action of an 'anti Xa' and also functions as an antithrombin.

22   D E
The major cardinal signs of acute inflammation were described by Celsus (30 BC-AD 38) as rubor (redness), tumor (swelling), calor (heat) and dolor (pain). To these is generally added functio leasa (loss of function) traditionally ascribed to Galen (AD 130-200).

23   A B D E
Chemicals mediate the vascular and cellular events that follow upon tissue injury, notably vasodilatation, increased capillary permeability and leucocyte emigration. Histamine is important in the initiation and early stages of inflammation. The kinins are biologically active polypeptides which are produced by the action of enzymes known as kallikreins on a kinin precursor called kininogen; bradykinin is probably best known. 5-hydroxytryptamine (5-HT or serotonin) is also released from mast cells and plays the same role as histamine. Prostaglandin production is stimulated by tissue damage and inflammation; PGE_1 and PGE_2 act as mediators and regulators of acute inflammation. Proconvertin is a clotting factor.

24   A B E
There are two major groups of phagocytic cells, the polymorphonuclear leucocytes of the blood, or microphages, and the mononuclear cells or macrophages. The latter may either circulate in the blood, when they are called monocytes, or may be fixed in the tissues, in which case they are called histiocytes; it is now established that tissue macrophages are derived from peripheral blood monocytes. It was previously assumed that macrophages were antibody producers, but there is now good evidence that

instead they act as antibody processing and presenting cells, which 'instruct' antibody production by lymphocytes. Macrophages may coalesce to form giant cells e.g. the fusion of epithelioid cells to form Langhan's cells in tuberculosis. They play no part in the coagulation process.

25   C D

The adrenal cortex produces three functional groups of steroid hormones. These are the glucocorticoids, principally cortisol and corticosterone, the mineral corticoids, mainly aldosterone, with small amounts of desoxycorticosterone; and the sex hormones, primarily the androgens, dehydroepiandrosterone androstene-dione and testosterone. Small amounts of oestrogens and pro-gesterone are also secreted. All these hormones are derived from cholesterol although the latter is not itself secreted by the adrenal, nor is it a hormone.

The secretion of cortisol is controlled exclusively by ACTH acting through specific cell surface receptors and the cyclic AMP system. Sex steroid secretion is also promoted by ACTH although other unknown factors must bring about the increase in androgen secre-tion which precedes puberty. ACTH also has a permissive effect on the zona glomerulosa ensuring adequate steroid precursors for aldosterone secretion. Control of aldosterone secretion however is determined by changes in the renin-angiotensin system. Over 98% of testosterone, 95% of cortisol and 60% of aldosterone in the circulation is protein bound.

Corticosteroids are degraded and conjugated with glucuronic acid in the liver but are excreted by the kidneys.

26   A B D

Polymorphonuclear leucocytes may appear in the immediate response to tuberculous infection although their appearance is very transitory and within 24 hours they are replaced by mononuclear macrophages. The ingestion of bacilli by those cells and the conse-quent dispersion of lipid throughout their cytoplasm leads to the development of epithelioid cells which are the most characteristic feature of tuberculous infection. Giant cells may arise from the fusion of several epithelioid cells and such giant cells with their multiple nuclei arranged peripherally are known as Langhan's cells. These various cell types along with a lymphocytic infiltrate form small follicles or tubercles; centrally such lesions undergo a form of coagulation necrosis or caseation resulting from the liberation of protein from the tubercle bacilli. Fibroblasts do not occur within the follicle although they may form a perifollicular capsule during the course of healing.

27 A C
Teratomas are tumours consisting usually of more than one germ layer; they may occur at any site in the body although the vast majority arise in the gonads. Congenital dermoids are inclusions of dermal tissue along the line of embryonic fissures, occurring especially in the midline; they may be attached to the external surface of the body (e.g. in the sacral region) or included within a body cavity (e.g. in the mediastinum).

28 A C E
A papilloma is a benign epithelial tumour whose cells cover finger like processes of stroma. A fibroma is a benign connective tissue tumour made up of fibroblasts and collagen fibres in varying proportion. A neurofibroma is a benign fibrous tumour of the endoneurium of cutaneous or deeper nerve trunks; the cutaneous form may be multiple (von Recklinghausen's disease), and both forms may progress to sarcomatous change.

The seminoma is a malignant testicular tumour, of seminiferous tubules. Multiple myeloma is a malignant tumour of bone marrow affecting specifically the plasma cells.

29 B C E
The cystadenoma, granulosa cell tumour, and teratoma may all occur in the ovary, being derived from neoplastic growth in epithelial, sex cord, and germ cell structures respectively.

The nephroblastoma and neuroblastoma are developmental tumours of kidney and nerve tissue respectively, occurring almost exclusively in early childhood and generally showing a sarcomatous appearance.

30 A C
Urinary calculi may consist of uric acid and urates (in approximately 8% of cases) calcium oxalate (in 60% of cases), cystine (in 2% of cases) and mixed calcium ammonio magnesium phosphate (in 30% of cases); the latter however are usually secondary to urinary infection.

Calculi in the biliary tract may be either pure cholesterol, pure bile pigment, or of mixed composition. Silicon is the most widely distributed element on the earth but it does not occur normally in the human body.

31   A B C E
An embolus is a 'foreign' material transported from one part of the circulatory system to another, whence it becomes impacted. The most usual form of embolus is a thrombus formed in the heart or blood vessel wall, which becomes detached. Other types of emboli include air (usually from iatrogenic causes), fat (often following fracture of a long bone), tumour (by direct invasion of the circulation by malignant cells, or by dissemination at the time of surgery), and amniotic fluid (following rupture of membranes especially during rapid labour). Urinary, biliary, or salivary calculi cannot enter the circulation, and therefore cannot form emboli.

32   A D
Aldosterone is produced by the cells of the zona glomerulosa of the adrenal cortex. It is secreted in response to increased levels of circulating angiotensin II. Renin is secreted by the juxtaglomerular cells of the kidney in response to decreased renal perfusion, decreased ECF volume or sodium depletion; it acts on the α_2 globulin angiotensinogen to produce angiotensin I, and a pulmonary converting enzyme subsequently produces angiotensin II, which in turn stimulates aldosterone release. Aldosterone is independent of plasma osmolality per se although ADH secretion is altered in response to osmotic changes induced by aldosterone. Although potassium loss is one of the effects of aldosterone secretion, potassium levels have no controlling influence on aldosterone. There is an oestrogen induced increase in plasma renin substrate in pregnancy; the increased sodium losses due to the increased GFR, in addition to the fetal demands for sodium also lead to an increase in plasma renin, angiotensin II, and aldosterone.

33   B C
Parathormone (pth) is secreted by the so-called transitional cells of the parathyroid glands; the thyroid C-cells produce calcitonin. The control of parathormone secretion is by alterations in the ionised calcium level in the blood, an increase in Ca^{2+} (other than from primary hyperparathyroidism) leading to a reduction in hormone output. Hypermagnesaemia also leads to a decrease in pth secretion although it is unlikely that this effect is of physiological significance. The effects of pth are to produce hypercalcaemia, hypophosphataemia, hyperphosphaturia and hypercalcuria and increased urinary hydroxyproline excretion; these changes result from increased bone resorption, decreased tubular reabsorption of phosphate and increased absorption of calcium in the gastrointestinal tract. Parathormone has no effect on the pituitary.

34   A C E

Prostaglandins are 20-carbon unsaturated fatty acids with a cyclo-pentane ring; although initially isolated from semen they have been shown to be present in most if not all organs of the body and to be implicated in a wide variety of physiological processes. Prostaglandin $F_2\alpha$ (Pg $F_2\alpha$) is shown to be present in increased amounts in the endometrium in the luteal phase of the menstrual cycle and may lead to spasm within the spiral arterioles. Increased Pg synthesis by the granulosa cells of ovary prior to ovulation has been postulated to lead to the release of collagenase, lysosomal enzymes, and plasminogen activator, all of which may play a part in the erosion of the superficial layers of the ovary overlying the dominant follicle. Pg $F_2\alpha$ has also been implicated in luteolysis. Pg synthesis from the decidua and myometrium is one of the mechanisms postulated to lead to the onset of labour; a similar effect may underlie the symptom of dysmenorrhoea.

Several prostaglandins have been manufactured and are commercially available.

35   D E

Cytotoxic drugs do not kill tumour cells directly but affect cell division and thereby cell proliferation. Alkylating agents such as cyclophosphamide transfer alkyl groups to biologically important cell constituents such as amino, carboxyl, sulfhydryl or phosphate groups whose function is then impaired. 5-fluorouracil is an antimetabolite which interferes with the synthesis of nucleic acids. Plant alkaloids such as vincristine and vinblastine produce mitotic arrest by binding to a cytoplasmic precursor of the spindle. Many of the antibiotics such as adriamycin bind selectively to DNA forming complexes that block the formation of DNA-dependent RNA. The precise mode of action of hormones is unknown but tamoxifen acts as an anti-oestrogen, not as an agonist.

36   B D E

Basal body temperature often drops by 0.1 to 0.2°C transiently around the time of ovulation followed by a sustained rise of 0.5 to 1.0°C which is maintained throughout the luteal phase. The plasma L.H. which surges to a peak around 12 hours prior to ovulation falls progressively during the luteal phase. Plasma progesterone secretion by the corpus luteum increases to a peak around 7-8 days after ovulation and as a result the endometrium undergoes a secretory change, and cervical mucus becomes more scanty, viscid, and cellular.

37 B E

HCG is a glycoprotein being composed of two amino acid chains designated α and β, both of which have carbohydrate residues which make up approximately 10-30% of the molecular weight. The α subunit is common to all the glycoprotein hormones, while the β subunit, is specific and therefore radio-immuno-assay (RIA) may be directed to this part of the molecule. HCG is produced throughout pregnancy being first detected by RIA within a week of ovulation and reaching a peak at around 10 weeks gestation. Because of the structural similarity between HCG and LH, a functional overlap also exists and HCG may be used in the treatment of ovulatory dysfunction, to stimulate ovulation and corpus luteum formation. The effects of HCG in pregnancy are on the corpus luteum itself, rather than on the uterus, and serve to maintain progesterone secretion until such time as the placenta is capable of autonomous steroid secretion. In excessive amounts, e.g. in trophoblastic tumours, lutein cysts may result.

38 A C D

The male primitive germ cells, the spermatogonia, are diploid, as are the primary spermatocytes; thereafter a reduction division occurs such that the secondary spermatocytes, spermatids, and mature spermatozoa are haploid with a chromosome complement of 23. FSH promotes spermatogenesis by a direct action on the seminferous tubules; LH promotes secretion of androgens by the Leydig cells and these, testosterone in particular, are important also in stimulating spermatogenesis. The total sequence of spermatogenesis (the formation of spermatids) and spermiogenesis (the formation of spermatozoa from spermatids) takes 65-75 days under normal circumstances. The process is however very sensitive to environmental changes particularly of temperature; the normal scrotal temperature is 1- 2.5°C lower than core temperature, and even slight elevation will impair sperm production.

39 B D

The normal secretion of prolactin by acidophil cells of the anterior pituitary is modulated by a 'prolactin inhibiting factor', probably dopamine, secreted by the hypothalamus. Bromocriptine acts as a dopamine agonist and therefore suppresses physiological or pathological secretion of prolactin at the hypothalamic level. It is thus indicated in hyperprolactinaemic states and may be used to suppress puerperal lactation (although in practice it is rarely necessary in this latter situation, except following stillbirth or neonatal death, where prevention or rapid resolution of breast engorgement is desirable). Bromocriptine is also used in acromegaly as an adjunct to surgery or radiotherapy since it has been shown to suppress growth hormone secretion also.

40   A E
The sulphonamides, tetracyclines, and chloramphenicol are primarily bacteriostatic drugs whereas the penicillins and aminoglycosides (incl. streptomycin) are bacteriocidal. The distinction is of some relevance in that two bacteriocidal drugs may be synergistic, and two bacteriostatic drugs may be so to a lesser degree, but combinations of bacteriostatic and bacteriocidal drugs may be antagonistic in some cases.

41   A E
Oxytocin is a polypeptide hormone (strictly an octapeptide, although described as a nonapeptide in some texts since it contains one cystine molecule, made up of two cysteine residues). It is secreted by cell bodies in the supra optic and paraventricular nuclei of the hypothalamus, and stored prior to release in the posterior pituitary. It is close in structure to antidiuretic hormone, being distinguished from it by only two amino acids, and there is functional overlap in that oxytocin has an ADH effect. The other more direct effects of oxytocin are on the uterus and myoepithelial cells therefore promoting milk ejection (but not formation) and uterine contractility; this latter effect is maximal in late pregnancy and is potentiated by oestrogens.

42   A C
Thyroxine, or tetra-iodothyronine, is produced by coupling of two molecules of the iodinated tyrosine derivative di-iodotyrosine. It circulates largely in bound form to the plasma protein thyroid binding globulin, thyroid binding pre-albumin and albumin, only 0.04% being in the free form. Among the biological effects of thyroxine are its stimulant effect on growth and development, both overall growth and maturation of specific tissues being effective. It leads to an increased oxygen consumption and heat production, as recorded by an increase in basal metabolic rate; brain, spleen, testis, uterus, and anterior pituitary do not increase O_2 consumption in response to increased thyroxine levels. Serum cholesterol is lowered in hyperthyroidism and raised in hypothyroidism.

43   A D
Cytotoxic drugs exert their effects predominantly on rapidly dividing cells and they may therefore affect fetal development and cause abortion or congenital malformation when used in the first trimester; this risk is greatest with folic acid antagonists such as

methotrexate and alkylating agents such as cyclophosphamide. Penicillin readily crosses the placenta but appears to be entirely safe for use in pregnancy. Heparin does not cross the placenta and is thus non-teratogenic. Testosterone may cause virilisation of a female fetus with clitoral hypertrophy and labial fusion if given to a mother in early pregnancy; other studies suggest an increased incidence of other congenital malformations including cardiovascular abnormalities, limb defects and neural tube defects. Barbiturates have been used as sedatives in pregnancy for over 50 years and although there have been sporadic reports of abnormality there is no convincing evidence of significant teratogenicity.

44 A B C
Escherichia coli and the other enterobacteriaceae including *Proteus sp.* and *Klebsiella sp.*, commensal in the gastrointestinal tract, commonly cause urinary tract infection of endogenous origin. *Clostridia sp.* although often gastrointestinal and vaginal commensals are not associated with such pathogenicity in the urinary tract. *Neisseria gonorrhoeae* is an intracellar organism affecting glandular epithelia such as the endocervix, rectum, and paraurethral and Bartholin's glands; it does not occur in the urinary tract.

45 B C E
Candida albicans is a fungus commensal in the human gastrointestinal tract. It is an opportunistic pathogen and host defences usually have to be weakened before infection occurs: diabetics, alcoholics, drug addicts, those with anaemias or leukaemias in addition to pregnant or pill-taking women are particularly prone to infection. The organism may be identified microscopically by the large budding yeast cells with long pseudohyphae; flagellae are not present. Culture of suspected specimens should be carried out on Sabouraud's medium. Nystatin, in the form of cream or pessary is usually effective treatment: failure may be due to reinfection from the bowel and oral treatment should be given concurrently.

46 C D
The gonococcus is a Gram-negative intracellular diplococcus which does not exist in an anaerobic form. Infection may have a bacteraemic phase with resultant gonococcal arthritis or endocarditis; the more usual sites of infection in the female however are the endocervix, endosalpinx, urethra, rectum, pharynx, and Bartholin's glands. Up to 1976 all strains were penicillin sensitive although since then increasing reports of β-lactamase producing, penicillin resistant organisms have appeared.

47 **A B E**
Tuberculosis of the female genital tract most commonly occurs by haematogenous spread following primary pulmonary infection. Whilst 10% of women with genital tuberculosis will have had previous pregnancies, subsequent infertility may be a feature in up to 70%. Tuberculosis of the lung and renal tract occurs with the same frequency during pregnancy as at other times.

The principles of antibiotic therapy for tuberculosis traditionally are that three drugs to which the organisms are fully sensitive should be used for 3 months, and thereafter only two drugs need be continued for a minimum of nine months. More recently regimens of shorter duration (6 months) have been advocated, but at least two drugs must be employed.

The degree of acid fastness of the various mycobacteria species varies; tubercle bacilli retain their red staining with carbol-fuchsin (Z-N staining) when challenged with 20% H_2SO_4.

48 **A C**
The total red cell mass, in the absence of iron supplementation, increases by around 18%; the increase appears to be approximately linear from the end of the first trimester up to term. The plasma volume increases by approximately 40% in healthy primigravid patients; this increase is greater in multigravidae, and in multiple pregnancy, and less in association with fetal growth impairment and pregnancy induced hypertension. The mean corpuscular haemoglobin concentration does not change significantly in normal pregnancy, or in folate deficiency. The mean red cell volume changes little in normal pregnancy; values less than 80 fl are highly suggestive of iron deficiency, the reduction in mcv occurring before any change in mchc. The total white cell count increases in pregnancy, due largely to an increase in neutrophils.

49 **A B**
Thyroid hormone binding proteins are increased by oestrogens, and thus in pregnancy and in combined oestrogen/progesterone oral contraceptive users the protein bound iodine (pbi) increases. Androgens cause a decrease in thyroid hormone binding proteins and thus treatment with androgens or increased protein losses as in nephrosis are associated with a fall in pbi. Drugs such as salicylates or hydantoins compete for binding sites on the proteins with thyroid hormones and therefore also cause a reduction in pbi.

50 **A C D**
Vitamin K exists in nature in two forms K_1 and K_2 both derivatives

of the cyclic structure naphthoquinone, which is fat soluble. Vitamin K is readily synthesised by *Escherichia coli* and other gastrointestinal commensals and hence primary dietary deficiency never arises in man. When long-term broad spectrum antibiotics are used the disturbance in bowel flora may lead to deficiency. Its main function is in formation of coagulation factors II, VII, IX and X by the liver; deficiency may therefore be associated with haemorrhagic phenomena especially in the premature newborn whose liver function may be immature.

51   A C D E
The Mullerian duct (paramesonephric duct) arises as a groove in the mesonephric ridge, lateral to the mesonephric duct. The groove becomes tubular by the fusion of the two edges of the invagination. The upper part forms the Fallopian tube and its cranial end remains open into the peritoneal cavity. The free caudal end of the Mullerian duct crosses the mesonephric duct and approaches the urogenital sinus. On the dorsal wall of the sinus the two ducts fuse to form the Mullerian cord which will become the uterus and cervix. The mesonephric or Wolffian ducts are concerned with epididymus and vas deferens formation in the male. The primitive urogenital sinus does receive the mesonephric ducts and is continuous along the mesonephric openings with the allantois. The lower part of the vagina may develop from canalization of the sinovaginal bulbs.

52   A
Amniotic fluid volume rises with gestation to around 36 weeks, volumes being approximately 30 ml at 10 weeks, 250 ml at 20 weeks, 750 ml at 30 weeks and 900 ml at 36 weeks; thereafter liquor volume falls slightly to around 800 ml at term. Up to midpregnancy the amniotic fluid has a composition similar to fetal extracellular fluid, and its volume is closely related to fetal weight. During the second half of pregnancy the fetal skin keratinizes and continuity between fetal extracellular fluid and the amniotic cavity is lost; fetal urine production then provides a large contribution to amniotic fluid volume, and hence the creatinine content progressively increases and osmolality falls with advancing gestation. Liquor alphafetoprotein level falls from 14 weeks to term.

53   A E
The term sex-linkage is virtually synonymous with X-linkage; the Y-chromosome appears to have few loci apart from those determining the male sex. The only documented Y-linked state is that of the 'hairy pinna'.

Congenital ichthyosis is an X-linked disorder associated with a steroid sulphatase deficiency (and hence may be associated with very low oestriol levels in pregnancy).

Hurler's syndrome is determined by an autosomal recessive gene, and achondroplasia by an autosomal dominant. Cleft palate, whether or not associated with cleft lip, seems to have a multifactorial inheritance pattern.

54　B C

The standard deviation of a series of observations is a measure of the extent of their spread about their mean. It is calculated from the mean and the number of observations but each individual observation must also be known.

$$s.d. = \sqrt{\frac{\Sigma\,(x-\bar{x})^2}{n-1}}$$ where
Σ = sum of all observations
x = indiv.obs.
$\bar{x}$ = mean obs.
n = number of obs.

It is used in several tests of significance but is not in itself a measure of significance. It is only meaningful for observations that have a normal, Gaussian distribution, and in such populations may be used to predict centiles e.g. mean $\pm$ 1 s.d. includes 68% of population therefore mean $-$ 1 s.d. is equivalent to the 16th centile and mean $+$ 1 s.d. to the 84th centile; the standard deviation is however not synonymous with a centile.

55　B

Arginine vasopressin, antidiuretic hormone, is produced by cell bodies in the supraoptic and para-ventricular nuclei of the hypothalamus and is stored and released from the posterior pituitary. It is an octapeptide (although having a cystine molecule, made up of two cysteine residues joined by a disulphide bond it is referred to as a nonapeptide in some texts). It increases the permeability of the distal tubule and collecting ducts to water and therefore increases reabsorption and decreases urine volume. Its release is controlled by changes in plasma osmolality and plasma volume, the osmoreceptors being in the hypothalamus although the location of volume receptors is uncertain. Deficiency of vasopressin causes the clinical picture of diabetes insipidus; alcohol inhibits vasopressin release.

56　A C D

The tidal volume is the amount of air inspired or expired with each respiration. The maximum volume that can be inspired beyond the tidal volume is the inspiratory reserve capacity. The total lung volume is the sum of the inspiratory reserve capacity plus the tidal volume and the functional residual volume.

The respiratory dead space is that volume occupied by gas which does not exchange with blood in the pulmonary vessels; it is therefore made up of the anatomical dead space of the trachea and bronchi plus the extra volume of the alveoli that do not contribute to gas exchange.

The vital capacity is the total amount of air that can be expired after a maximum inspiratory effort (i.e. the inspiratory reserve plus tidal volume plus expiratory reserve capacities, it is the latter which is described in part E).

The functional reserve capacity is the expiratory reserve plus the residual volume i.e. the amount of gas in the lungs at the end expiratory position. Both the expiratory reserve and the residual volume are reduced in pregnancy and hence the functional reserve is reduced by around 500 ml or 20% of non-pregnant values, at term.

57   B C E
Gastrin is not an enzyme but a polypeptide hormone secreted by cells in the pyloric antrum. Protein, alcohol and caffeine all stimulate secretion, although carbohydrate and fats have a lesser effect. The major effect of gastrin is to stimulate acid secretion from the parietal cells in the glands of the body of the stomach; (mucus neck cells also occur in the glands of the body which secrete mucus and intrinsic factor). Histamine is also a potent stimulant of gastric acid secretion and indeed it has been suggested that gastrin may act by causing histamine release from mast cells in the gastric mucosa.

58   A C
Acetylcholine has been shown to be the transmitter substance released by preganglionic fibres of both sympathetic and parasympathetic systems. Postganglionic fibres of the parasympathetic system secrete acetylcholine as well, although with a few exceptions (e.g.sweat glands) sympathetic post-ganglionic fibres have nor-adrenaline as their transmitter substance. Within the brain, in addition to acetycholine and nor-adrenaline, 5- hydroxytryptamine, histamine, dopamine, γ amino-butyric acid, and prostaglandins may all act as neurotransmitters.

Impulses only pass in one direction across synapses which are more sensitive to hypoxia and chemical agents than nerve fibres.

59   A B C D
The muscle of the ciliary body in the eye, the bronchial walls, and the gall bladder all contract in response to acetylcholine release

from post-ganglionic fibres of the parasympathetic nervous system. The arrectores pilorum, the smooth muscle of hair follicles contract in response to nor-adrenaline release from sympathetic fibres. Sweat glands, although innervated through the sympathetic nervous system have acetylcholine as their transmitter at post-ganglionic nerve endings.

60   A B C E

Folic acid is a water-soluble vitamin of the B group. It is widely disseminated in both plant and animal products although the main dietary source in man is green leafy vegetables. Unlike vitamin B_{12} which requires intrinsic factor for absorption it has no mediating absorptive mechanism and is assimilated throughout the small intestine. It is converted to the coenzyme tetrahydrofolinic acid which is important in the transfer of one-carbon units in purine synthesis; deficiency leads to a megaloblastic macrocytic anaemia.

RECOMMENDED BOOKLIST

There is no specific reading list for the College examination; the following list, whilst certainly not exhaustive, contains texts which have been suggested as background reading by the College, in addition to others which we feel candidates may find useful during their preparation.

Anatomy:
Gray H. **Gray's Anatomy.** 37th ed. 1989 Longmans.
Ham A. W. **Histology.** 9th ed. 1987 Lippincott.
Last R. J. **Anatomy: Regional and Applied.** 8th ed. 1990 Churchill
Livingstone.

Embryology:
Sadler T. W. **Langman's Medical Embryology.** 6th ed. 1990 Williams and
Wilkins.
Wendell-Smith **Basic Human Embryology.** 3rd ed. 1984 Pitman.

Physiology and Endocrinology:
Ganong W. F. **Review of Medical Physiology.** 14th ed. 1989 Lange.
Hall R. **Fundamentals of Clinical Endocrinology.** 4th ed. 1989
Churchill Livingstone.
Hytten F. E. Chamberlain G. V. P. **Clinical Physiology in Obstetrics.**
2nd ed. 1990 Blackwell.
Passmore R. Robson J. S. **A Companion to Medical Studies, volumes 2
& 3. 2nd ed. 1980 Blackwell Scientific.**

Genetics:
Emery A. **Elements of Medical Genetics.** 7th ed. 1988 Churchill
Livingstone.
Thompson J. S. Thompson M. W. **Genetics in Medicine.** 4th ed. 1986
W. B. Saunders.

Microbiology:
Duerdon. **New Short Text Book of Microbial and Parasitic Infection.** 1990
Edward Arnold.
Gillies R. R. **Bacteriology Illustrated.** 5th ed. 1984. Churchill Livingstone.
Sleigh J. D. Timbury M. C. **Notes on Medical Microbiology.** 3rd ed. 1990
Churchill Livingstone.

Pharmacology:
Goodman L. S. Gilman A. **Pharmacological Basis of Therapeutics.**
8th ed. 1990 Macmillan.
Graeme-Smith D. G. Aronson J. K. **Oxford Textbook of Clinical
Pharmacology and Drug Therapy.** Revised ed. 1990 Oxford.
Hawkins D. **Drug and Pregnancy.** 2nd ed. 1987 Churchill Livingstone.
Laurence D. R. **Clinical Pharmacology.** 6th ed. 1987 Churchill Livingstone.

Pathology:
Hoffbrand, Pettit **Essential Haematology.** 2nd ed. 1984 Blackwell Scientific
Publications.
Hughes-Jones N. C. **Lecture Notes in Haematology.** 5th ed. 1991 Blackwell
Scientific Publications.
Walter O. B. Israel M. S. **General Pathology.** 6th ed. 1987 Churchill
Livingstone.

Statistics:
Bradford-Hill A. A. **A Short Textbook of Medical Statistics.** 2nd ed. 1985
Hodder and Stoughton.
Swinscow T. **Statistics at Square One.** 8th ed. 1983 B.M.A.

General Basic Sciences Texts:
Chard T. Lilford R. **Basic Sciences for Obstetrics and Gynaecology.**
3rd ed. 1990 Springer-Verlag.
Dewhurst, de Sweit, Chamberlain **Basic Sciences in Obstetrics and
Gynaecology.** 1986 Churchill-Livingstone.
Phillipp E. Barnes Newton M. **Scientific Foundations of Obstetrics and
Gynaecology.** 3rd ed. 1991 Heinemann.

MCQ REVISION INDEX

Each item in this index is followed by a number which refers to a specific question in one of the practice exams, i.e. 3.27 refers to Practice Exam 3 question number 27.

PASTEST MEDICAL BOOKS

	ISBN
MRCP Part I Revision Book Edited by B. Hoffbrand DM FRCP	0 906896 03 7
MRCP Part I Practice Exams Edited by P. Ackrill MB ChB FRCP	0 906896 16 9
MRCP Part I MCQ Pocket Series : Ed. R. Hawkins	
Book 1 : Cardiology and Respiratory Medicine	0 906896 18 5
Book 2 : Neurology and Psychiatry	0 906896 19 3
Book 3 : Gastroenterology, Endocrinology and Renal Medicine	0 906896 23 1
Book 4 : Haematology, Infectious Diseases and Rheumatology	0 906896 24 X
MRCP Part I MCQs with Subject Summaries Edited by P. O'Neil BSc(Hons) MB ChB MD MRCP	0 906896 55 X
MRCP Part I Explanations to the Royal College blue booklet of MCQs	0 906896 31 2
Medicine International MCQs: Book 1 (Out of Print)	0 906896 04 5
Book 2	0 906896 15 0
Book 3	0 906896 65 7
Oxford Textbook of Medicine MCQs : second edition	0 906896 22 3
MRCP Part II Revision Book (with colour plates) Eva Lester MBBS MRCPath	0 906896 08 8
MRCP Part II Preparation for the Clinical Exam Julian Gray MA MB BS MRCP(UK)	0 906896 45 2
MRCP Part II Pocket Series : Ed. R. Hawkins	
Book 1 : Cardiology and Respiratory Medicine	0 906896 37 1
Book 2 : Gastroenterology, Endocrinology and Renal Medicine	0 906896 42 8
Book 3 : Haematology, Rheumatology and Neurology	0 906896 47 9
MRCP Part II General Medicine (A4 size) Colour slides, data and case histories etc.	0 906896 27 4

MRCP Part II Paediatrics (A4 size) Colour slides, data and case histories etc	0 906896 32 0
MCQs in Psychiatry Grant, McDonald & Bell	0 906896 35 5
MRCOG Practice Exams Part I P. Hilton MB BS MRCOG	0 906896 25 8
The DRCOG Examination S. Mellor, M. Read, S. Bootle and J. Sandars	0 906896 61 4
MRCGP Practice Exams : Revised edition John Sandars MRCP MRCGP	0 906896 30 4
Learning General Practice J. Sandars and R. Baron	0 906896 41 X
Short Notes for the DCH J. R. Blackburn and G. Curtis Jenkins	0 906896 70 3
Primary FRCS Practice Exams Edited by Forsling and Chambers	0 906896 17 7
Primary FRCS Revision Book Forsling, Abraham and Chambers	0 906896 07 X
FCAnaes Part I Practice Exams Ingram and W. Aveling	0 906896 26 6
FCAnaes Part II Practice Exams M. Forsling and L. Bromley	0 906896 75 4
PLAB Medical Practice Exams Parashchak and Ibrahim	0 906896 20 7
PLAB English Practice Exams Joy Parkinson BA	0 906896 21 5
Postgraduate Medical Training in the UK: Edited by C. Quarini MSc	0 906896 66 5

FOR OUR FULL CATALOGUE OF CURRENT
MEDICAL TITLES AND PRICES PLEASE WRITE TO:

PASTEST, FREEPOST
KNUTSFORD, CHESHIRE WA16 7BR
Tel: 0565 755226

Notes